Educating Pupils with Autistic Spectrum Disorders

About the Book

'Martin Hanbury is full of enthusiasm and extremely knowledgeable.'

Cathy Mercer, National Autistic Society

Martin Hanbury's book is an invaluable tool for developing positive and enduring learning relationships in inclusive classroom environments. It draws on his extensive experience of working with children with autistic spectrum disorders.

Written for educators in both mainstream and special provision schools, as well as teachers who are new to the field or those who are working in isolation from other specialists, the book gives practical advice on how to employ appropriate teaching and learning strategies.

The book includes:

- an overview of autism and how it affects learning

- suggestions for established, effective strategies and interventions

- advice on how to select the appropriate strategies for individual pupils

- INSET materials to use in staff meetings and on INSET days

- tried and tested ideas for successful lessons

- handy hints and checklists

- a glossary

- a selection of photocopiable material ready for the classroom.

Additional photocopiable resources are available to download from the PCP website (**www.paulchapmanpublishing.co.uk/resources/hanbury.pdf**).

Martin Hanbury is the Headteacher of Landgate School, Bryn – a school for children with autism. He has worked with people with autism for over twenty years in a range of roles including carer, classroom assistant, teacher and school manager.

Educating Pupils with Autistic Spectrum Disorders

A Practical Guide

Martin Hanbury

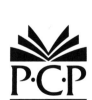

Paul Chapman Publishing

London · Thousand Oaks · New Delhi

Paul Chapman Publishing
A SAGE Publications Company
1 Oliver's Yard
55 City Road
London EC1Y 1SP

SAGE Publications Inc
2455 Teller Road
Thousand Oaks, California 91320

SAGE Publications India Pvt Ltd
B-42 Panchsheel Enclave
PO Box 4109
New Delhi 110 017

Library of Congress Control Number: 2004112795

A catalogue record for this book is available from the British Library

ISBN 1 4129 0122 4
ISBN 1 4129 0228 2 (pbk)

Typeset by Pantek Arts Ltd, Maidstone, Kent
Printed in Great Britain by Cromwell Press, Trowbridge, Wilts

This book is dedicated to
Pat and Antony Hanbury

Thanks to Liz Blackburn, Paul Blair, Penny Cullen, Sean Cullen, Andrew Knott, Debra Knott, Jenny Partington, Gillian Reilly and John Reilly

Contents

Acknowledgements

Those of us lucky enough to work with children learn something new each day. Generally, it is the child who teaches us and our progress as practitioners depends largely on our ability to respond to what we have learnt. I hope I have listened to the children I have worked with and would like to thank them for all they have taught me. Equally, the families and carers of these children are a special group of people. Their resilience, creativity and focus on their children's needs have been both inspirational and informative. Again, I would like to thank them all.

I have faced the challenges we encounter in education alongside colleagues whose skill and commitment has deepened my faith in humankind. I must thank, in particular, the staff of Inscape House, Salford and my colleagues at Landgate School, Wigan who have supported and encouraged my work with patience, sensitivity and good humour.

Several colleagues made unique contributions to the good practice shared in this book. I would like to thank especially Graham Birtwell (Peterhouse School, Southport), Keith Cox (Inscape House, Salford), Anne Murray (Radlett Lodge School, Hertfordshire), Tony Newman (Stanley School, Wirral), Lucy Wood (Aspin House, Southampton) and Melanie Wilkinson (Ashton, Leigh and Wigan P.C.T.) for their hard work and positive attitudes towards this project.

Similarly, I have benefited enormously from the advice and judicious culling suggested by my editor, Jude Bowen. This book has been an adventure; without her guidance it may have been more of a ramble.

Finally, I must thank Theresa for creating the space for me to work in and Megan, Timothy, Patrick and Francis for their patience.

Foreword

Over 30 years ago I was invited to an interview at a school for children with autism. How I got to this point is a long story and I shall not bore the reader with it here. I searched the libraries and bookshops of west London for information on these children and emerged with three books: a volume of various articles by Leo Kanner, *The Siege* by Clara Claiborne-Park and *The Empty Fortress* by Bruno Bettelheim. The interview took place in half term and having been offered the position I turned it down as, from what I had read, there was no way I could work with these children. The then Principal, Lusia Arendt, was a very determined lady and paid for me to come back and spend a day in the school. The day became over 17 years and I had the privilege of being the third Principal of the Sybil Elgar School.

At that time I had the strong belief that it was a good thing that children with autism did not read what is written about them. Since those early days there has been a gradual increase in books on autism and, more recently, a dramatic surge, seeming to accompany the so-called explosion in autistic spectrum disorders, in provision across all elements of education. As Barry Carpenter said at the Equals Conference in 2000: 'In whatever area of education you work, there is one thing you can be sure of – in the future you will be providing for more children with autism.' Clearly this impacts on those on the shop floor – the teachers, assistants and SENCOs.

This book is one of those gems in the literature available for providing strategies to aid the hard-pressed professional. From the clear description of the history of autism and the delineation of various theories and approaches, it launches into established and tested strategies in working with children with autism. Most importantly, it starts with the premise that autism is not an 'in-child' problem. This book is an invaluable tool kit. Had this book been available some 30 years ago, perhaps my early steps into this field would have been less faltering.

I leave the last words to a young man with autism:

> School days provide the earliest opportunity for social contact, and yet I remember those days with trepidation ... If only I had had the right sort of professional support at school while on school premises, life would have been so much easier. Someone to make me less oblivious of the impression which I was giving other pupils, and to give strategies (Thomas Mader, a person with an ASD).

Mick Connelly
Blackpool Education and Children Service
2005

Prologue

Feelings remain clearer than events. Memory has a place for emotion, sealed against the lapses of time. Fresh, preserved, it surges through you as it did at the moment it first marked you. So I can see him now, knees curled into his ribs as if yet unborn, the side of his face pressed against the soft plastic of the seating, humming the tune to Thomas the Tank Engine.

Then, one day, there was some news. He was leaving. He was going down South somewhere, to a school for pupils who had something called autism. 'What's autism?' I asked. 'It's what he's got', I was told.

That was my introduction to the field of autism, twenty years ago and somewhat accidental. Those first years working with children with autism remain profoundly influential. The feelings I had then of intrigue and confusion, of feeling totally inadequate and yet being unable to think of anything else I'd rather do, are as pertinent and fresh today as they were then. And that is because, in the field of autism, each child you meet is a new beginning, a new starting point, a new learning curve. Why? Perhaps it is because no matter how many people with autism you've met, *you* are the first *you* they've met. To a person with autism, that matters.

Introduction

This book grows from a need, an urgent need, to address the daily challenges facing practitioners in the field of autism. The National Autistic Society's (**NAS**) report *Autism in Schools: Crisis or Challenge* (Barnard et al., 2002) presents a picture of practitioners, in all sectors of education, addressing increasingly complex issues against a backdrop of fundamental change and reform. The lack of a national autism register and the absence of sound, large-scale epidemiological research means that reliable statistics relating to the prevalence of autism are not available, further contributing to the challenges faced by school managers and LEA officers in planning and developing appropriate provision. The difficulties faced, therefore, pervade every tier of the educational process from the chalk face to the DfES and no single panacea can be prescribed for a problem which is both endemic and systemic. There are, however, individualised strategies for particular situations which can be effective and enduring, and the purpose of this book is to support the process of developing and customising these approaches for the specific situations in which practitioners are working.

Despite the lack of robust statistical information, there remains a strong consensus amongst professionals that the prevalence of autism in schools is increasing, a consensus which is endorsed by several key indicators. In their report, the NAS (Barnard et al., 2002) cite figures produced by the Medical Research Council which estimated that 1 in 166 of children under eight experienced Autistic Spectrum Disorders (ASDs). This coupled with teachers' perceptions that 1 in 86 pupils have needs related to ASDs and schools reporting that 1 in every 152 pupils has a formal diagnosis of ASDs strengthens the anecdotal evidence provided by many practitioners. The discrepancy between the current rates of ASDs reported in primary and secondary schools, with primary teachers reporting prevalence three times higher than that of their secondary colleagues, prompts the NAS report to ask:

- Is the higher rate at primary level a result of higher levels of awareness and better diagnosis?
- Are there missing children at secondary school level?
- Does this give credence to those who claim that we are witnessing an 'autism epidemic'?

(Barnard et al., 2002: 6)

Whatever the case may be, for the practitioner one thing is clear: there is an increasing number of pupils who are, or will be, identified as autistic and who will require specialised, highly skilled input. Each of these youngsters represents a unique position on the autistic spectrum and provision should reflect the variety and richness which these children bring to our nurseries, schools and colleges.

Yet responding to such diversity remains fundamentally problematic for two key reasons. Firstly, the field of autism is expanding at a rate which cannot be served by the experienced and qualified practitioners currently available. Secondly, there are a variety of factors, beyond the control of the practitioner, which profoundly affect the learning of the child with autism. Those of us involved in the day-to-day education of pupils with autism, can often feel helpless when confronted by obstacles we can do nothing about.

However, as practitioners, there is one key area we can affect – *ourselves*. The quality of our practise can be profoundly influenced by improving our knowledge and skills, and it is the intention of this book to support practitioners by drawing on the wealth of experience and expertise currently available in the field and sharing that with all colleagues.

This reservoir of good practice has been hard won. Children with autism are a uniquely challenging group; challenges which arise from the very essence of autism as defined within the **triad of impairments** by Lorna Wing (1996). Pupils with autism display a number of traits which deviate significantly from expected learning pathways and they rarely learn in the neat, incremental ways on which our educational system is based. Children with autism can sometimes appear to suddenly know something or seem to instantly master a skill without any attention to the learning which forms its foundation. Equally, there can be inexplicable deficits in areas of apparent strength or a rapid deterioration of established skills.

Children with ASDs can strike at the heart of what it is to be a practitioner. Good, child-centred practitioners are motivated by the strong and enduring relationships they form with children. Children with autism often find forming relationships problematic and can remain distant and apparently disinterested in the adults around them for prolonged periods. These features can be seen to undermine the basis of the pupil–teacher relationship and consequently erode a person's confidence, self-esteem and sense of self. Therefore, to work with these children requires a person who can skilfully accommodate being selfless, yet be remarkably thick-skinned; who is empathic whilst remaining determined; a person who is, to coin a phrase, a 'soft rhinoceros'. And it is this type of person who can make all the difference for the child with ASDs; a unique practitioner for a unique child.

The purpose of this book is to support the practitioner through practice, starting with the simple maxim to:

> Start by doing what is necessary,
> then what's possible and suddenly,
> you're doing the impossible.

(St Francis of Assisi)

Chapter 1

Autism: An Overview

- Provides a brief history of autism including discussion of theories of causation, diagnostic criteria and changes in prevalence.

- Presents current understanding of the condition through the conceptual models of the triad of impairment, mind-blindness, difficulties in executive function and difficulties in central coherence.

In the early nineteenth century, the French physician J.M.G. Itard, seen by many as the father of special education, offered the first documentary evidence of an individual who we might reasonably describe as autistic. Itard's study of Victor, a non-verbal child discovered in the woods around Averyon, provided the first methodical study of autism and presented an account of the attempts to educate the child, particularly in respect to the development of language skills.

Later in the nineteenth century, Henry Maudsley proposed that children with distinctively abnormal behaviour patterns might be suffering from childhood psychoses, a revolutionary idea at the time as it introduced the concept of the child as a complex psychological being. In the early part of the twentieth century, various other writers including De Sanctis, Potter and Earl described many features that we would recognise as associated with autism, although they used terms such as 'childhood schizophrenia' and 'catatonia'. Importantly, none of these descriptions attempt to define a coherent group or recognise commonalities which might constitute a syndrome. However, knowledge and learning was coalescing, gradually converging to a particular point of understanding.

KANNER AND ASPERGER

It is in the seminal work of Leo Kanner (1943) that we first find the word autism applied to an identifiable group of youngsters who shared common characteristics representing a unique and specific condition different from any other childhood conditions. A year later, Hans Asperger (1944) working in wartime Austria, reported a group of adolescents who, although of average or above average intelligence, shared the same features of social ineptitude, inflexible thought patterns and idiosyncratic use of language. In the immediate aftermath of war, it was Kanner's work which received wider publicity and engaged the scientific community in further studies of causation and definition.

Kanner's initial work focused on 11 children, eight boys and three girls, who at the time he was writing were all under 11 years old. Kanner identified in these children many of the features of autism we would recognise today including:

- the inability to relate themselves in the ordinary way to people and situations

- excellent rote memory

- language – which the children did not use for the purpose of communication

- insistence on sameness.

(Kanner, 1943: 242–5 *passim*)

Moreover Kanner recognised that despite the variation amongst the individual children he was studying, there existed sufficient common characteristics to denote a specific condition. He says:

> The eleven children (eight boys and three girls) whose histories have been briefly presented, offer, as is to be expected, individual differences in the degree of their disturbance, the manifestation of specific features, the family constellation, and the step-by-step development in the course of years. But even a quick review of the material makes the emergence of a number of essential common characteristics appear inevitable. These characteristics form a unique 'syndrome,' not heretofore reported, which seems to be rare enough, yet is probably more frequent than is indicated by the paucity of observed cases.

(Kanner, 1943: 241–2)

In articulating this notion of a singular condition comprised of a range of manifestations, Kanner prefigured the complexity of the condition which was to gradually emerge over the coming decades.

The circumstances of war entailed that Asperger remained unaware of Kanner's paper and his use of the term 'autistic' when publishing his own work. Asperger used the same label to describe four children aged between 6 and 11, who showed marked difficulties in social integration despite apparently having adequate cognitive and verbal skills. Asperger drew a distinction between his patients' lack of social contact and the withdrawal of children with schizophrenia by highlighting the fact that children with schizophrenia displayed a progressive withdrawal, whereas his patients showed this aloofness from the outset. Asperger stressed that impaired social interaction was the defining feature of his patients' condition and provided a comprehensive list of symptoms and features including:

- difficulties in interpreting non-verbal communication, such as facial expressions and body movements
- peculiar use of language
- obsessive interests in narrowly defined areas
- clumsiness and poor body awareness
- behavioural problems
- familial and gender patterns.

(Asperger, 1944)

In many respects Asperger's original work had little influence on the field of autism until the 1970s. Then, as notions about autism evolved to incorporate a broader spectrum (Gillberg, 1985; Wing and Gould, 1979), so the group associated with Asperger began to be included in the debate. Because of the distinctions between the two original groups studied, it became usual to describe people of lower cognitive ability as classically autistic, or as experiencing Kanner's autism, whereas more able individuals were seen as experiencing Asperger's Syndrome.

It is important to note at this point that the relationship between autism and Asperger's Syndrome remains a controversial arena for discussion (Cohen and Volkmar, 1997). The basic standpoints are:

- Kanner's autism and Asperger's Syndrome are part of a spectrum of associated disorders known as autistic spectrum disorders. People with Asperger's Syndrome represent a high functioning group within the spectrum.

- Asperger's Syndrome is distinct from other conditions. High functioning autism is not the same as Asperger's Syndrome; there are qualitative differences in the condition.

Studies that have attempted to identify criteria which discriminate between autism and Asperger's Syndrome have yielded mixed results. We must recognise that our understanding of autism is still at a very early stage in its evolution and consensus over the precise demarcation of groups will remain problematic for some time to come. As educators, our primary concern does not lie with diagnostic distinctions but rather with the features of the condition(s) which adversely affect a pupil's ability to learn; our focus must remain here.

CAUSATION

Early ideas of causation were obscure and confusing. It must be remembered that Kanner was a psychiatrist operating in the climate of psychoanalytic thinking which had become predominant in the 1940s. Consequently, ideas about the cause of autism began to form around theories of parenting and, in particular, the role of the mother in nurturing the child. Kanner takes time to comment:

> This much is certain, that there is a great deal of obsessiveness in the family background ... One other fact stands out prominently. In the whole group, there are very few really warmhearted fathers and mothers.

> (Kanner, 1943: 250)

Whilst Kanner notes the likelihood of a biological factor in the causation of autism, the spirit of the age seized upon his notion that autism was caused by cold, mechanical parenting which resulted in emotional damage in otherwise healthy, intelligent children. The work of Bettelheim was particularly influential in compounding and perpetuating this error which led to a generation of mothers, cruelly tagged as 'refrigerator mothers', suffering the terrible burden of not only having a severely disabled child but also being blamed for their child's disability.

As time passed, the clear overlap between autism and learning disability prompted many professionals in the field to question Kanner's assertions that this condition was psychogenic. But it was not until 1964 and the publication of Rimland's work, showing that autism was a biological disorder and not an emotional illness, that the myth was dispelled. Even so, significant damage had been done and the vestiges of early misconceptions about causation continued for many years.

Today, the question of causation remains unclear with research focused in three key areas, namely:

- psychology

- neurology

- genetics.

Each of these fields may be characterised as follows:

- **Psychology** – relating to an individual's cognition, perception and understanding. Research has focused on language, memory, spatial awareness, sensory perception, social awareness and empathic awareness.

- **Neurology** – relating to the dysfunction of particular structures of the brain and the neurochemicals which transmit information within the brain. The commonality of symptoms across the spectrum has led researchers to investigate a unique underlying neurobiology.

- **Genetics** – relating to the inherent characteristics which make up an individual. It is generally accepted that genetic factors play a major role in the aetiology of autism. Current research has focused on determining the chromosomes and genes that are responsible for causing the brain dysfunction associated with autism. However, evidence would seem to indicate that causation does not lie at a single location but rather within complex matrix of genetic factors.

Whilst investigations in each of these key areas are essential for furthering our understanding of autism, the differing perspectives held by researchers in each discrete field can lead to confusion. Furthermore, definitions of the term 'cause' may vary significantly amongst researchers just as the phenomena being studied may be wide-ranging. Consequently, there are a variety of different, sometimes conflicting, theories of causation.

For our purposes as educators, it may well be necessary to take a pragmatic, though somewhat simplistic, view on this issue. Based on what we know, it is reasonable to see autism as a *behaviourally defined developmental disorder which is the result of neurological dysfunction caused by, as yet, undetermined factors likely to include a strong genetic influence.*

If we ask of a particular individual, 'What causes this person's autism?', our answer lies along a complex chain of events defined by several levels of causation. A geneticist answering the question will refer to the aetiology, a neurologist will reference brain pathologies and a psychologist will point to the developmental issues affecting the person. Our understanding, as educators, is best informed by taking account of this complexity and attempting to integrate each level of causation in order to produce a picture of the whole child.

A further point to consider is that at each level there may be a number of possible causes. Therefore, there may be a number of genetic factors, a variety of possible brain pathologies and a range of developmental impairments which lead to the spectrum of behaviour we term autism. Indeed, the fact that there are perhaps many permutations of causation may well account for the breadth of the spectrum and the 'fascinating peculiarities' (Kanner, 1943: 217) of each unique individual with autism.

DIAGNOSIS

Whilst theories of causation fluctuated over the years, the complex nature of autism determined that agreement on a definitive set of criteria for the condition would be problematic. Kanner had provided vivid, evocative descriptions of the children he reported in 1943 but he provided no operational diagnostic criteria. However, working with Eisenberg in 1956, an attempt was made to provide diagnostic guidance for the condition he had identified via five key features, namely:

1   a profound lack of affective contact with other people

2   an anxiously obsessive desire for the preservation of sameness in the child's routines and environment

3   a fascination for objects, which are handled with skill in fine motor movements

4   mutism or a kind of language that does not seem intended for inter-personal communication

5   good cognitive potential shown in feats of memory or skills on performance tests.

Kanner also stressed the need for the age of onset to be no later than thirty months. This diagnostic basis became known as 'classic autism' or 'Kanner's autism' and was condensed into these two fundamental features:

1   a profound lack of affective contact

2   repetitive, ritualistic behaviour, which must be of an elaborate kind.

However, autism is a shifting condition which seems to shrink from definition, reforming itself each time an attempt is made to capture its essence. As with all true enigmas, the more we know, the less we understand, the closer we come to holding it, the further away it seems to slip. Whilst Kanner and Eisenberg's criteria might have been regarded as a starting point, it was soon to be superseded by a succession of other diagnostic criteria, each endeavouring to provide clarity in what was proving to be an increasingly obscured field.

Mildred Creak (1964) led a working party which defined nine key features. These were:

1   sustained impairment of interpersonal relationships

2   unawareness of personal identity

3   pre-occupation with particular objects

4   striving to maintain sameness

5   acute anxiety produced by change

6   abnormal perceptual experience (hearing and vision)

7   failure to develop speech beyond a very limited level

8   distortion of movement

9   some learning difficulty, but some islets of particular skills or abilities or knowledge.

This list, known as 'Creak's Nine Points', represented the first attempts at a sys-temised method for diagnosis. As knowledge increased, so did the debate around defining this apparently diverse yet strangely uniform group. In 1978 Michael

Rutter proposed four criteria which he derived from a combination of Kanner's descriptions and his own clinical experience:

1 impaired social development which has a number of special characteristics out of keeping with the child's intellectual level

2 delayed and deviant language development that also has certain defined features and is out of keeping with the child's intellectual level

3 'insistence on sameness' as shown by stereotyped play patterns, abnormal preoccupations or resistance to change

4 onset before 30 months.

In 1980 the American Psychiatric Association published the third edition of *Diagnostic and Statistical Manual of Mental Disorders*, known generally as DSM III, which considered infantile autism as a subgroup of associated conditions termed 'pervasive developmental disorder'. Following a series of revisions to include the more subtle features of autism, a system for diagnosis was published in DSM IV (A.P.A. 1994). This framework forms the basis for diagnosis currently used by many paediatricians.

The other system of classification used by many clinicians is the World Health Organization's *International Statistical Classification of Diseases and Related Health Problems*, or ICD. The edition known as ICD 10 (1992) was the first edition that did not consider autism as a form of psychosis, marking an important point of arrival for the field of autism. ICD 10 classifies autism as one of several pervasive developmental disorders ensuring that the basis for diagnosis, agreed upon by each of the major systems used by clinicians, is developmental.

However, despite the adoption of these systems, the issue of diagnosis remains extremely problematic. This is because autism is defined by what we can see, that is, an individual's behaviour. There is no clear 'marker' which can be clinically obtained and therefore diagnosis reflects the opinion of the diagnostician following observation and interviews with care providers. Whilst for many children, the nature of their condition lends itself easily to diagnosis, there are many children for whom the picture is not clear. This might be for several reasons including:

1 The manifestation of those features cited as diagnostic criteria in DSM IV and ICD 10 is inconsistent; appearing in certain contexts and apparently not in others.

2 The child's condition is complicated by other difficulties such as profound and multiple disabilities, severe learning difficulties, mental health problems or generally poor health.

3 The child's developmental history is not fully known, therefore diagnostic tools reliant on developmental checklists are compromised.

4   The symptoms of autism may change with age and developmental progress – nevertheless, autism remains a lifelong condition.

In cases such as these the child may remain without a diagnosis for long periods of time. The effect of this can be significantly damaging with youngsters not able to access appropriate care and education and parents remaining in a diagnostic limbo. However, we must recognise the difficulties faced by diagnosticians given the broad-ranging spectrum embraced by the condition and the complexity of the individuals within that spectrum.

PREVALENCE

The range and variety of diagnostic models which have become prominent over the years, dictates that determining a precise figure for the population of individuals with autism is very difficult. Since Kanner's original work, many important large-scale studies have taken place, such as Lotter (1966) Wing and Gould (1979) and Gillberg (1984). However, as the definition of autism has been fluid, so the populations studied have varied significantly (Wing, 1993). For example, Lotter's study used Kanner's classic descriptions of the condition and estimated the prevalence of autism as 4 to 5 people in every 10,000. However, using a broader interpretation of a spectrum of autistic disorders, Wing and Gould arrived at a figure of 20 per 10,000. In a study of mainstream schools in Sweden Gilberg, Steffenburg and Schaumann (Gillberg et al., 1991) broadened the definition even further and concluded that 71 in every 10,000 pupils displayed social impairments of an autistic type.

Recent studies have suggested that early estimates of the prevalence of autism were conservative. Research from the 1990s to the present day shows significant annual rises in the prevalence of autism with as many as 60 people per 10,000 reported by some researchers (Wing and Potter, 2002). The reason for this marked increase is as yet unproven, but may be accounted for by the following factors:

- changes in diagnostic criteria

- the evolution of a concept of a wide spectrum of autistic disorders

- increased awareness and therefore identification of the condition

- possible environmental causes.

Whichever factor, or combination of factors, is in operation, the fact remains that we are finding increasing numbers of children with autism in our schools, an issue which must be urgently addressed.

MODELS OF AUTISM

As educationalists, our attention should be focused on endeavouring to understand how the condition affects the way a child with autism perceives the world around him or her. To this end, we need to consider several important models of autism in order to begin to understand the experiences of the young people we are working with. Perhaps the best known model is centred on Wing's notion of the triad of impairments (Wing, 1996). This model, based on clinical experience and extensive research, recognises core deficits in the areas of:

- social communication

- social interaction

- imagination.

and crucially indicates that the severity and manifestation of these fundamental impairments will vary significantly

> ... we found that all children with 'autistic features', whether they fitted Kanner's or Asperger's descriptions or had bits and pieces of both, had in common absence or impairments of social interaction, communication and development of imagination. They also had a narrow, rigid, repetitive pattern of activities and interests. The three impairments (referred to as the 'triad') were shown in a wide variety of ways, but the underlying similarities were recognizable.

(Wing, 1996: 25)

The strength of Wing's model is that it is flexible enough to embrace the full range of the autistic spectrum whilst remaining conceptually coherent and focused on these three core deficits. A diagrammatic representation of the triad might look something like Figure 1.1 in which the circle A represents impairment in social communication, circle B impairment in social interaction and C impairment in imagination. Autism occurs where all three circles intersect.

Figure 1.1   The Triad of Impairments

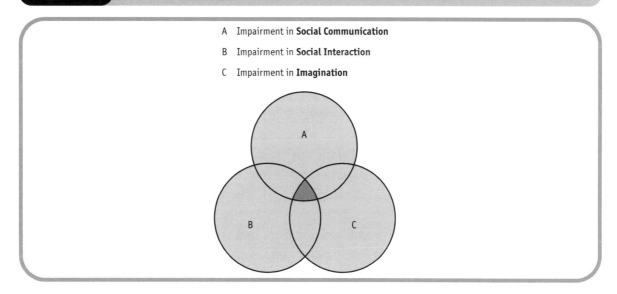

A   Impairment in **Social Communication**

B   Impairment in **Social Interaction**

C   Impairment in **Imagination**

For educators in both mainstream and specialist settings, Wing's model allows us to see each child's condition uniquely. Whilst it is necessary for all three impairments to be present, the degree to which each of these components affects the person with autism varies from individual to individual. For some people, one element of the triad may be particularly marked, whilst others may show significant difficulties across two components and hardly any in the third. For certain people, the overall impact of the triad may be profound, whereas for other people the affects may be comparatively manageable. The infinite possible combinations and permutations of the triad accounts for the huge breadth of the autistic spectrum and the great variety found within it.

A further benefit of this model for educators is that it enables us to reflect upon our practice and the environments in which we practise from the perspective of a person with impairments in these three crucial areas. Schools are essentially *social* settings which operate through the medium of *communication* and depend upon an *imaginative* negotiation of an infinitely complex and unstable environment. If a person experiences fundamental problems in these key areas, it is little wonder that, regardless of their cognitive potential, schools are difficult places to be.

Another important idea to consider is **mind-blindness** (Baron-Cohen, 1990, 1995) which is based on the view that people with autism lack a 'theory of mind'. Simon Baron-Cohen argues that a theory of mind, that is the ability to appreciate the mental states of oneself and other people, is a prerequisite to effective functioning in social groups. The argument continues that as the human race evolved and societies became increasingly complex and subtle, so the capacity for greater 'social intelligence' increased in order to allow us to process information about the behaviour of others and respond accordingly. This 'adaptive' behaviour is usually evident in children from the age of four upwards. However, children with autism seem to lack the ability to 'think about thoughts' (Happe, 1994) suggesting they are impaired in specific, but crucially, not all, areas of socialisation, communication and imagination. As educators we might see the lack of a theory of mind emerging as an inability to grasp the social etiquette of the classroom, an apparent lack of feeling towards peers or a failure to share the excitement that other children may feel. Quite simply, children with autism cannot get inside other people's heads. Therefore their understanding of others is profoundly limited.

Early developmental difficulties, which may be associated with mind-blindness, include problems in infants showing joint attention skills (Sigman et al., 1986), usually evident by 14 months of age, and the later failure of being unable to engage in pretend play (Leslie, 1987), which normally emerges between 20 and 24 months old. As a theory of mind is not usually fully developed before four years of age, difficulties in these two areas may be seen as early indicators of subsequent problems. In the normally developing child, sharing attention with another person shows an awareness of the separateness of another person's thoughts. Joint attention skills incorporate monitoring or directing the focus of attention of another person through pointing, gestures and gaze-monitoring and are invariably absent in the child with autism. Similarly, the ability to engage in pretend play depends upon having a concept of another person's mental attitude (Cohen and Volkmar, 1997) towards an object or activity, that is, an awareness that they are pretending too. The failure of this skill to emerge prefigures difficulty in the realm of appreciating other people's thoughts, that is, mind-blindness. For educators, these early signs may be evident in pre-school settings as infants and children appear to be disinterested in activities which captivate other children and fail to engage in the shared fun of pretend play.

The third model of which educators need to be aware is that which is related to difficulties people with autism have in the area of **executive function**. Executive function is the mechanism which enables us to move our attention from one activity or object to another flexibly and easily. It allows us to plan strategically, solve problems and set ourselves objectives so that we can control our behaviours in planned and meaningful ways (Norman and Shallice, 1980). The absence of such a mechanism determines that all our actions are controlled by the environment in response to cues and stimuli, leading to apparently meaningless activity. Without an executive function, actions and behaviours compete for dominance in a disorganised and inconsistent manner leading to an inability to plan and execute goal-generated behaviour. In a school setting, this emerges as highly distractible behaviour coupled with a dependence upon ritual and routines and an apparent disregard for the school timetable or the completion of tasks.

A fourth concept which educator's need to consider is **central coherence theory** (Frith, 1989). This notion relates to our natural impulse to place information into a context in order to give it meaning. It is usual for human beings to take an overview of things, to look for the 'big picture' and assimilate the detail into that whole. However, people with autism tend to focus on the detail rather than the whole, picking out the minutiae rather than understanding the big picture. It has been found that people with autism show superior abilities in finding the 'embedded figures' from pictures (Shah and Frith, 1983) and they are better able to recognise the identity of familiar faces from a part of the picture than their non-autistic peers (Campbell et al., 1995). Similarly, children with autism fail to use context clues when reading (Happe, 1997), often mistaking the meaning of homographs, for example, tear as in drop, for tear as in paper. Whilst some of these examples refer to superior ability, this superiority denotes a failure to appreciate the whole and accounts for the piecemeal way in which people with autism acquire knowledge and the unusual cognitive profile presented by many people with autism. Educators may detect the lack of central coherence in the narrowed interests of children with autism in the ways in which pupils with autism are often unable to generalise skills, or the way in which they may display areas of relative strength, known as islets of ability.

The models portrayed above represent a part of the conceptual framework which underpins current thinking in the field of autism. It is important to consider that this framework is constantly being added to and reshaped as our knowledge of the condition increases. However, the ideas discussed above are well founded and remain established as significant agents in our understanding of autism, and are of particular use to the educator engaged in the challenge of developing the learning of the child with autism.

EDUCATION

As understanding amongst professionals developed, the particular educational needs of children with autism became increasingly apparent. However, the controversies over diagnosis and causation, combined with the sheer breadth and variety of the autistic spectrum, meant that developments within the field of education were slow and stuttering. Commenting on the situation in the UK, Elgar and Wing reported that:

> Early childhood autism is not specified in the list of categories of handicapped children requiring special educational treatment. However, the Department for Education and Science has indicated to Local Education Authorities that if a child is diagnosed as autistic or psychotic he should receive at least a trial of education.
>
> (Elgar and Wing, 1975)

So much for entitlement for all then! These sentiments may seem to be cast in another age and yet, in terms of educational history, they come from the relatively recent past. Indeed, reflecting on this statement, I realised it was written at a time when I was at school and other children of my generation, due to their autism, were considered ineducable. At this time, just under half of the known autistic population of school age were in Subnormality Hospitals, some of which had schools attached but many children received no teaching at all. A small number of children were accepted into mainstream schools, but it was observed that these children, whilst often progressing well in the earlier years, tended to encounter problems as they moved towards the later years of primary school and into secondary school.

However, there were movements within the field driven largely by parents' groups, professionals and the National Society for Autistic Children, later the National Autistic Society. In 1960, Dr Mildred Creak had requested that two children with autism be admitted to a unit at Hollymount, Wimbledon, run by Surrey County Council. More children with autism were gradually admitted until in 1965 the school became the Lindens School, Epsom. In the same year, the National Society for Autistic Children opened its first school in Ealing with Sybil Elgar as the Headteacher.

Other than providing specialist provision and all the benefits that may accrue from that, the absolutely crucial contribution made by Barbara Furneaux at Hollymount and Sybil Elgar in Ealing, was to dispel previous assumptions about the learning of children with autism. Before their work it had been believed that these children required treatment prior to education. However, through the efforts of these pioneers, it was shown that education was a crucial part of their general development and that for children with autism, treatment and education were indeed one and the same thing. That this important breakthrough appears obvious to us now is a testament to the enduring quality of the achievements of this pioneering group of educators and places us forever in their debt.

Chapter 2

The Impact of Autism on Learning

- Presents the impact of autism on learning as consisting of three waves affecting the whole child.

- Discusses how this impact affects learning, the family, professionals and peers.

As practitioners working with children with autism, we must ask ourselves:

What are the main obstacles to learning faced by children with autism?

The answer to this question is not a simple list of the impairments associated with the condition. The answer lies in an awareness of the affect of these features on the child's learning. The quality of our practice depends on how we move from *knowing* about the condition towards *understanding* the impact of these impairments on the child.

This ability to think beyond the textbook, to integrate knowledge, understanding and empathy, is vital because there is no such thing as a 'textbook' child with autism. Whilst every child is unique, children with autism have a unique uniqueness. Consequently, we cannot follow a prescribed 'one-size-fits-all' formula but need to develop approaches which address the needs of each individual.

Autism can be seen as having three 'waves' of impact on the child's learning which radiate outwards from the child. These three waves are:

1   the affect of the condition itself

2   the behaviour which occurs as a result of the condition

3   the attitudes which form as a consequence of the child's behaviour.

The first of these incorporates those primary features of autism which directly affect the child's learning, such as communication difficulties, rigidity, sensory issues or problems with organising thoughts. These in turn cause a second wave of impact which is characterised by the behavioural features associated with autism. These behavioural issues trigger a third wave of impact which is defined by the relationships and attitudes the child forms with the world around them. This model is illustrated in Figure 2.1.

Figure 2.1   **Autism: Three Waves of Impact**

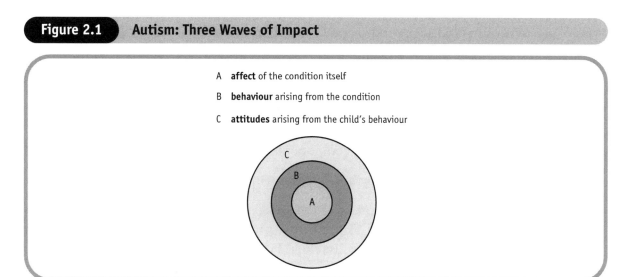

A   **affect** of the condition itself

B   **behaviour** arising from the condition

C   **attitudes** arising from the child's behaviour

THE AFFECT OF THE CONDITION

This level of impact is an immediate consequence of the child's autism. Although the impact of the condition is inevitable, it can be obscured by other factors which accumulate around the child. For the practitioner to make a positive contribution to the learning of the child, it is necessary to develop an understanding of the child which is rooted in the nature of the condition. This is achieved not only through increasing our knowledge but also by evolving a 'perceptive sympathy' that enables the practitioner to see through to the child and the impact of autism on the child's learning.

Social Impairment in the Classroom

Walk into any classroom, in any school, and what immediately strikes you? Essentially, that you have entered an infinitely complex and sophisticated social environment. Most of us have found classroom society difficult to cope with at some point in our lives and this should be no surprise. Classrooms can be confusing places with subtle and inconsistent social rules, shifting allegiances and power constantly changing hands. As an antidote to this, children adopt roles within the culture of the classroom, whether it be the joker, the chameleon, the sporting hero, the swot, the social butterfly or the bully. We all look to perform some function in the social mechanism because we have an innate understanding of the social role expected of us and that we expect of others.

However, if you have autism, how do you negotiate this daunting passage of your life? It is difficult enough for those without ASDs, so how much harder must it be for the child whose innate understanding of society is impaired; for the child who doesn't see what everybody else sees or think the way that everybody else thinks? Consider the fundamental obstacles to a child's social functioning brought about by impairments in the ability to:

- read social situations

- understand social codes and expectations

- interpret facial expression and body language

- appreciate other people's feelings

- engage other people through social 'devices' (smiles and small talk)

- determine the important components of social interaction

- organise actions into orthodox patterns.

It is arguable that for almost any other special need, the classroom only becomes disabling when a demand to perform a given task is made. For the child with autism, the classroom itself is disabling. For many children with autism, disability begins at the door.

Communication Difficulties

Another inescapable feature of any classroom is that it is a communication-dense environment. The classroom is alive with a myriad of communicative acts, some hidden, some obvious, some deliberate, many unintentional. This pertains to all classrooms in mainstream, special or specialist schools. Indeed, it applies to all environments in which children learn.

So, for the child whose communication skills are impaired, this rich, fast-flowing stream of communication may seem more like a tidal wave of 'sound and fury, signifying nothing'. Consider the difficulties in effectively engaging in the communicative environment of a classroom from the perspective of a child who is unable to:

- comprehend much of what is said to him or her

- adequately express thoughts, needs, emotions, wishes

- discriminate which language is intended for him or her

- discern a person's tone of voice and what it might mean

- understand humour, idiom, sarcasm

- initiate communication

- recognise the need to reciprocate communication.

Impairments in communication place the child with autism in an alien world which is confusing, frightening and unintelligible. The spoken word flies past, peppered with sudden unexplained outbursts. Non-verbal communication is a cacophony of frowns, furrows and jerks which is meaningless and often threatening.

Inflexible Thinking in a Playful Environment

When children play, they exercise that most important of human faculties, the ability to think adaptively. They become increasingly skilled in the exploration of their thoughts and are soon tasting tea in empty plastic cups, hearing teddy read and seeing elephants in banks of clouds. And whilst all of this is lovely to watch and join in with, it serves an evolutionary purpose. From these playful groundings, human beings learn to adapt to the chaotic and to formulate flexible structures, which organise their lives and yet allow for the quakes and shakes of the real world.

In many ways schools are working examples of evolutionary processes, of adaptation to the environment, of survival. From the earliest years in nurseries children are required to think with a sophistication that seems beyond their years. In any classroom, in any school, we will encounter a number of situations which demand that the child thinks imaginatively, flexibly and adaptively. Children gather on the floor for story-time, drive diggers through the sand, write as if they are Victorian child labourers, design maps of non-existent cities, carry messages to teachers they have never met, choose subjects to suit careers they have not yet embarked on. All of this requires a fantastic imaginative effort. Not to mention the disputes and difficulties, the taking of turns, the avoiding of trouble and the very necessary daydreaming. Again all this is imagination dependent, necessitating flexible thinking and adaptive behaviour.

But, if your autism disables you in the social slalom of the classroom, it is likely that you will either rush headlong downhill, unable to deviate from your course, or perhaps, not even start the race by opting out entirely. Consider the 'unseen world' of the classroom from the point of view of the child who is unable to:

- engage in pretend play

- project themselves into future situations

- comprehend a world outside their experiences

- access elements of the curriculum which rely on imagination

- understand deception

- think how others might think or feel how others might feel.

The difficulties caused by impairment in the realm of imagination are significant and far reaching. If we consider play as the foundation of learning, then impairment in a child's ability to engage meaningfully in play presents fundamental obstacles to that child.

BEHAVIOURAL ISSUES: FEAR, FLIGHT AND FIGHT

Autism is a 'behaviourally defined condition' (Charman and Care, 2004). There is no chromosomal marker, no physiological feature which tells us a child has autism. It is only by observing the child's behaviour that we can say that the child has ASDs and only by analysing that behaviour further can we develop strategies to meet the child's needs.

Fear

For children with autism, fear can be a dominant and often overpowering state of being. This can be seen as a direct consequence of severe difficulties in interpreting the world around them, in understanding what is happening to them or is going to happen to them. Naturally, if your ability to learn is restricted by the primary impact of the condition you experience, then more things remain unknown to you, consequently there are more things to be afraid of. Whereas, for most children encouragement from adults or peer pressure leads them to experience new things, for the child with autism the value of adult praise or the shame of losing face means very little. There is, therefore, little incentive to step into new territory.

Equally, if you perceive things in different ways to others, either because of sensory problems or because of the way your brain processes information, then you may well learn to be afraid of many things that other people are not fearful of whilst remaining unafraid of many things which are a danger to you. This may manifest itself as the child who sees no peril in darting across the busy dual carriageway and yet finds walking down the school corridor absolutely petrifying. Furthermore, fear breeds fear, so that associated objects become objects of fear themselves. The child who is scared of the supermarket because it is packed with strange people, noises and smells, develops a fear of the coat he is put in to go to the supermarket because he comes to learn what putting that coat on might mean. Subsequently, he develops a fear of coats of any type and refuses in the depths of winter to wear anything more than a T-shirt.

The consequence of such fear is that, in addition to the difficulties the child faces due to autism, there is a layer of fear and tension which can suffocate their learning and enjoyment of life. This capsule of fear is both important and necessary to the child and any attempts to draw the child from it must be considered as well as gradual. However, in order to enable features of the primary impact to be adequately addressed, it is vital that this layer of fear is dissolved.

Flight

Flight enables us to escape danger. In everyday life it helps us avoid uncomfortable situations with a range of subtle and sophisticated strategies. For the child with autism, flight is often an effective and well practiced defence mechanism.

However, as a pattern of behaviour, flight is invariably incompatible with the context the child is operating in. Within the classroom flight can manifest in several distinct ways, namely:

- running away

- refusal

- self-absorption

- obsession.

These behaviours may occur alone, in combinations, simultaneously or in a sequence, often a predictable series. Given the breadth of the autistic spectrum and the broad range of backgrounds and personalities involved, we may encounter a child whose initial response to demands is to run out of the classroom or dive under the nearest table. We might know of children who skilfully turn every topic of conversation towards their own particular interests or children who are apparently locked into flickering their fingers centimetres from their eyes. Though varied, each of these is a form of escape, a way of displacing the discomfort of the here and now with a form of behaviour which the child is master of and the outcome of which is within the child's control.

As practitioners, we must recognise that the flight behaviour is functionally significant for the child and our approach towards reducing the behaviour must be informed by the child's need to escape situations they find difficult. However, as with addressing a child's fear, it is only when we can engage the child that we can positively affect their learning.

Fight

Whilst by no means a necessary consequence of autism, there are associations between autism and aggressive behaviour which are the result of the frustrations and fears people with autism experience. It is usually the fight response which has the most immediate affect on the context in which the child with autism finds him- or herself and, is therefore, the response which is most hastily addressed. This is unfortunate given the fact that, invariably, the need to fight emerges if other levels of need have not been adequately understood and addressed. Consequently, we deal with the crisis rather than those factors which lead to the crisis.

For the child with autism whose needs are not adequately addressed, fighting becomes an effective and rapid means of getting those needs addressed. For those people with autism who experience significant learning difficulties, the capacity to develop other, more appropriate, strategies for meeting those needs is very limited. As a result, the child becomes increasingly dependent upon fighting in order to meet their needs and narrows the already limited range of strategies further in an ever decreasing spiral.

For some people with autism, this decline into aggressive and damaging behaviour has resulted in tragically restricted and oppressed lives, foreshortened by the consequences of their behaviour, such as self-injurious behaviour, physical trauma or medical intervention.

ATTITUDES TO AUTISM

This level of impact occurs as a result of the interaction between people with autism and others. It is the area of impact which we can most readily affect by increasing our own personal knowledge of the condition and sharing this with colleagues across all sectors.

Parents

Working closely with parents and families is essential for effective practice in the field of autism. Children with autism are complex and enigmatic (Frith, 1989) and no single person can be expected to design and implement an uniformly effective learning programme for such children. Consequently, liaison with parents is of paramount importance at every stage of the child's progress. Practitioners need to be guided by policies based upon well-founded practice and supported by senior managers whose organisations are open and honest.

Working with parents requires practitioners to be aware of the 'journey' parents may well have endured before the relationship is established. Depending upon the age of the child and the severity of the condition, parents may be experiencing a range of different emotions, including:

- grief – parents whose child has been recently diagnosed with autism are often at an early stage of adjusting to the news. This adjustment includes an indefinite period of grief during which parents may suffer from denial of the condition, depression or guilt.

- anger – this may be directed at services which they feel have failed their child or the attitudes of other people towards their child.

- anxiety – this can be focused on issues of the past, the present or the future and may involve concerns not only about the child with autism but also regarding siblings, partners and other family members.

A person's response to these emotions will vary significantly and produce a range of attitudes including:

- cynicism – parents whose experiences are dominated by a failure of services to support their child and family will naturally doubt that any professional is able or willing to provide that support.

- optimism – for some people, the start of their relationship with a dedicated practitioner will be seen as a new opportunity to improve matters for their child and family. They will draw on the knowledge of previous failures to shape a positive future for their child.

- defensiveness – collaboration with parents always carries a danger of intrusion and it is wise to exercise caution and invite collaboration rather than foist it upon people. Many parents may be distrustful of professionals who might be perceived as wanting to run their lives.

- openness – where an atmosphere of trust and mutual respect has been nurtured, parents are able to share information about their child enabling a whole picture of the child to emerge.

- isolationism – many parents describe their child's condition as disabling the whole family. Some parents report that their social life and their relationships with their extended family are severely affected and that they feel isolated and alone. This, in turn, can lead to distrust and extremely low self-esteem resulting in parents attempting to go it alone as they feel support will not be forthcoming.

- collaboration – if individuals have access to networks of other parents of children with autism, then it is possible to forge positive and fruitful relationships within these groups. People understand one another's difficulties and work together towards a common purpose.

Each of these attitudinal states can be seen to describe polar opposites. Commonly, it is a combination of a person's character, their experiences of services and the quality of support around them that shapes their attitudes. As practitioners we usually inherit people's attitudes. Our aim should be to foster attitudes which are at the positive end of the continuum.

Peers

Experienced practitioners in the field of ASDs often struggle to understand the way in which pupils with autism act or are uncomfortable with the behaviour some pupils with autism display. It is not surprising, therefore, that many of their classmates will be confused or disturbed by the actions and patterns of behaviour of their peers with autism.

For some children this lack of understanding may result in a refreshing acceptance of the child with autism for the person they are. However, some children may be fearful and this may result in ostracising, bullying or mocking the child with autism. These attitudes create a matrix of difficulties for the child with an ASD which exacerbate their already significant impairments in forming peer relationships. For example, a child who has problems with initiating social contact may find that on attempting to interact with his peers his endeavours are rejected, perhaps quite cruelly. Consequently, the incentive to attempt further interactions diminishes, reducing the opportunities for the child to practise and develop his skills, thereby establishing a vicious, ever decreasing, circle of isolation.

For many children with autism, the older they become the wider the gap between them and their peers grows. This is due, in part, to the increasing pressures of conformity which their peers experience as they approach adulthood and the need the majority of us have to belong to the group. Children with autism tend not to care for groups and are therefore excluded from the smaller units of friendship which might be appropriate to their needs.

Professionals

In many ways, a positive attitude towards pupils with autism is directly related to a person's understanding of the condition. Working with youngsters with ASDs is not easy; there is much about the condition which professionals can find de-skilling. For example, children with autism can be reserved, aloof, seemingly uninterested and dismissive of our best efforts. They can appear not to care about their peers or about their relationship with us as educators. This goes to the heart of what we do; as educationalists we pride ourselves on the ability to stimulate, to inspire, to build enduring relationships with children. If this is rejected, we are left with nothing to define us. It is, perhaps, a form of defence that can cause many professionals to see the child with an ASD as rude, unmanageable and beyond the scope of their talents.

A result of this is that many professionals are at best wary of working with children with ASDs and at worst openly hostile. Often this is rationalised as seeing the child as detrimental to the greater good of the school or class or presented as the school being unable to meet the child's needs given the environmental restrictions. Such standpoints may have validity in certain contexts. However, the increasing prevalence of the condition and the momentum behind the inclusion agenda will challenge these standpoints and drive change in these contexts.

Professionals must be supported in developing their knowledge and understanding of autism in order to enable them to address the needs of pupils with ASDs. Whilst the pressures to achieve this are significant, there are increasing opportunities for professionals to develop their understanding and knowledge of the condition and a variety of ways in which this might be achieved.

Chapter 3

Sharing Positive Attitudes Towards Pupils with Autism

- Suggests ways in which positive attitudes towards pupils with autism can be promoted by increasing people's understanding of the condition.

- Provides strategies to support practitioners in sharing knowledge with colleagues including **INSET** materials.

Part of our work as practitioners involved with pupils with autistic spectrum disorders is to promote and sustain positive attitudes towards children with autism. We can achieve this by addressing the third level of impact on the child's learning; namely, attitudes arising from the child's behaviour. This level of impact presents us with opportunities for immediate gains. In this area we are largely dealing with issues of sharing knowledge and understanding, in winning hearts and minds. This is undoubtedly a challenging objective which should not be underestimated. However, it is an accessible challenge in which the key factors are related to time and resources, as oppose to those 'within child' factors which will be encountered at the other levels of impact.

WORKING WITH OTHER PROFESSIONALS

A professional's attitude towards pupils with ASDs is directly related to their knowledge and understanding of the condition. Consequently, there is a need to develop systems and means by which knowledge and understanding about ASDs are shared with other colleagues. Understandably, we are in competition with a multitude of other demands on professionals and, therefore, need to promote information in an accessible and manageable form which is tailored to the context they are working in. The depth of knowledge required might lie on a continuum from awareness to expertise determined by the role they perform. Colleagues whose only contact with pupils with autism is during break-times or assemblies will need a different level of understanding to those colleagues who may share the same teaching space. Similarly these colleagues' needs will differ again from those people primarily responsible for the teaching of youngsters with ASDs.

Responding to this continuum of professional development need, our training portfolio might include:

- informal approaches
- INSET days
- outreach
- accredited courses
- resources.

Each of these depend upon practitioners within the field promoting the cause of pupils with ASDs in a positive and proactive manner. Of the many myths which surround autism, the belief that working effectively with pupils with ASDs is somehow arcane and open only to the weird and wonderful, is amongst the least helpful. As practitioners in the field, we must show colleagues that our practice is attainable to anyone who is committed to good practice and is willing to learn. Essentially, we must show other practitioners that, like themselves, we are working with children – children that need specific approaches – but still children.

Informal Approaches

Some of the most effective professional development takes place over cups of coffee. Share your work with your colleagues in the staffroom, over lunch on training days or at staff meetings and briefings. Above all, share your enthusiasm, present your work as attainable and your pupils as accessible.

Suggestion Box

Encourage colleagues to visit your classroom or school in order to observe your practice. Ensure that you have planned adequate time for discussion after the observations. Base your discussions on the impact autism has on the child, the strategies you use to address this and the progress the child is making as a result of this. You might structure their observations by giving them a checklist of issues to consider whilst they are observing. Invite colleagues into your workplace before they have a crisis. Increase their knowledge before major difficulties arise.

NB: It is in the nature of practitioners to want to get involved in the activity, to be hands on. However, in the field of autism, observation is a crucial component of practice. Insist that any professional visitor simply sits still and watches for a significant proportion of the time they spend with you. If necessary, velcro them to the chair!

Observation Checklist

1. What do you notice about the child's learning environment?

2. Does the pace of work differ from that of your practice?

3. How is language used?

4. What strategies are used to support understanding?

5. How would you characterise the interactions between child and adult?

6. What barriers to learning do you think the child may be experiencing?

7. How might you adapt your practice to meet this child's needs?

8. How engaged in the adult directed activities is the child?

9. How does the child indicate his/her needs?

10. What does the child seem to find rewarding?

Please photocopy this checklist, adapting it as necessary to the context in which you are working and the nature of your relationship with the person observing.

Educating Pupils with Autistic Spectrum Disorders © Martin Hanbury, 2005

INSET Days

The competition for INSET space is fierce and growing fiercer with each new DfES initiative. Training for colleagues must be accessible and context driven. At this level of input, most people will want to know how to address issues in their own practice rather than become expert in the field. A template and supportive materials for an INSET session are available in the appendix to this chapter (see Developing Practice for the Pupil with Autism). Once again, adapt these to the context whilst ensuring that you engage colleagues in a critical reflection of their practice in relation to the needs of the pupil with autism.

Outreach

Outreach takes many forms and is different things to different people in differing contexts. However, a general view would be that it involves supporting a child by sharing specific skills and knowledge, germane to the needs of the child. Successful outreach is characterised by the seven Cs, namely:

1 clarity

2 consensus

3 contract

4 child-centred

5 credible practitioners

6 consistency

7 collaboration.

This can be expressed as clear agreements between all parties involved in the project, arrived at via consensus, defined by a mutual contract and focused entirely on the needs of the child. Outreach must be delivered by credible specialists supporting the work of organisations with consistency in terms of the knowledge shared, the persons involved and the regularity of contact. Effective outreach is essentially collaborative, involving committed practitioners sharing expertise rather than one party 'doing' outreach to another.

Accredited Courses

There are a number of valuable and respected providers throughout the country. We are in the privileged position in the UK of having several centres whose work is internationally regarded and who offer a variety of modular courses which can stand alone or be combined into higher qualifications. Access to these courses is increasingly being regarded as a prerequisite to high quality practice for youngsters with autism. Information regarding the range of commended courses can be obtained from the National Autistic Society.

Resources

Always at a premium, appropriate resources are essential for people looking to work effectively with youngsters with ASDs. Resources may include a well developed library relating to issues in autism, software and facilities for producing bespoke materials for pupils, communication aids, cause and effect toys, and particular areas of your classroom or school, such as a soft-play area or a multi-sensory room. Sharing resources with colleagues enables them to trial items with children without having to waste money. Another noticeable phenomenon is the way in which people tend to listen much more attentively when resources are on offer!

NURTURING HOME–SCHOOL RELATIONSHIPS

For any child, the quality of the relationship between home and school has a profound affect on their learning. For a child with autism, this relationship is especially important in order to ensure effective communication and enable consistency across settings. Positive relationships between parents and practitioners are characterised by the following key elements:

- approachable practitioners

- openness, honesty and trust

- sharing ideas

- records of contact,

each of which must be continuously monitored and explicitly valued.

Approachable Practitioners

First impressions count for a lot. If parents are put off by their initial contact with practitioners or organisations it is hard to regain the trust and respect which are the lifeblood of any successful relationship. Approachability depends to some extent on a person's nature, however, there are strategies which can be adopted to ensure that an individual or organisation is as approachable as possible.

Suggestion Box

- Make a concerted effort to welcome parents into your school or classroom. Structure this so that learning is not disrupted.

- Make a point of contacting parents to give good news of their child's achievements, celebrate their successes. Avoid only ever speaking to parents about problems.

▶

- Offer to visit the child's home. Seeing the home context will increase your understanding of the whole child. Be aware that some parents may find this intrusive and in some circumstances it might be prudent to visit with another colleague.

- Try to establish a space within your school which the parents can consider their own. Create a learning resource within this space, for example, a parent library and information point.

- Parent workshops focused on issues related to autism can be both supportive and encourage parents into the school.

Openness, Honesty and Trust

These three elements are inextricably linked and mutually reliant. The last of these, trust, is the ultimate aim but is not attainable without the first two components. Trust can be hard to win if parents' previous experiences with professionals have been negative. It is doubly important in such cases to be explicitly open and consistently honest. At times there will be the need to discuss difficult and sensitive issues; avoiding such issues will damage your relationship with parents whilst inept handling of the situation will ruin the relationship completely. Take time to plan carefully what you will say and how you will say it. Record everything that is discussed and share these minutes with parents. Where necessary include other colleagues in order to support your interpretation of the issues that are discussed.

Sharing Ideas

As practitioners we have much to learn about the children we work with. They are typically complex and present unique characteristics which challenge our understanding and patterns of practice. We may hope to develop expertise, yet it is the child's parents who are the experts, that is, experts with regard to their child. The opportunity to share ideas allows us to combine expertise with experts' views. Such opportunities may vary in scale from informal discussions between one parent and one practitioner to conferences involving many interested parties. Whichever medium is chosen to share ideas, it is crucial to engender an ethos in which every person feels their ideas have value, that their perspectives have importance. Depending on the context you are working in, you may need to state this explicitly in order to encourage people who may be intimidated by professionals or suffering from low self-confidence due to the difficulties they are encountering with their child.

Suggestion Box

- Offer a programme of parent workshops for your parent group. In a mainstream setting, you may only have one or two families for whom these workshops are relevant. In this case, try to collaborate with neigbouring schools to form a cluster focusing on issues in autism.

- In the first instance, invite parents to a coffee morning and during this ask parents to identify issues on which they would like to focus.

- Devise a series of regular meetings addressing each issue in turn.

- Try to deliver the workshops in a variety of ways in order to suit both the content of the workshop and the range of learning styles within the parent group.

- Engage outside speakers for some of the workshops in order to widen perspectives.

Records of Contact

We live in an 'evidence-based' age, a time when we are required to record almost every professional action or decision process. Maintaining and sharing records of contact with parents provides a basis for mutual understanding as all parties have a common record to refer to when seeking clarification or planning ahead. A well-maintained, well-written home–school diary can act as a voice for the child with autism and an invaluable source of ideas and suggestions between parents and practitioners. A log book of significant telephone conversations between parents and practitioners provides a record of issues which have been discussed offering support where necessary.

PEER RELATIONSHIPS

Sharing a class with a child with autism cannot be easy; even, perhaps especially, if you are a child with autism yourself. Consequently, we should be looking for as many ways as possible to equip children who are in the same class as pupils with autism with the skills that will enable them to cope with this demanding situation.

The development of these necessary skills is based on an expanding understanding of autism amongst pupils, centred around:

- increasing awareness of the condition

- developing understanding of individuals' needs

- recognising achievement

- deflating peer pressure.

Progress in any one of these areas leads to progress in one of the others; progress in all leads to an increased understanding amongst all pupils.

Before embarking upon any form of information-sharing with pupils, it is crucial to determine the extent to which the child with autism is aware of their condition and the degree to which they might want that knowledge shared. This is an ethical minefield which can only be successfully negotiated through extensive consultation with the pupil, the child's family, colleagues and organisations dedicated to the field of autism. In certain circumstances it may be necessary to postpone initiatives to share knowledge about autism; what is in the best interests of the child with autism must determine this decision.

Increasing Awareness

A continuous programme of information about autism will increase the knowledge and understanding of the condition amongst the child's peers. The nature of this programme will vary according to the learning ability and maturity of the pupils in the class. However, certain features will be universal. For example, there will be the need to introduce the concepts, if not the terminology, of those components of the condition which account for much of the behaviour that will be observed. Similarly, children may benefit from learning about the prevalence of autism in their community in order to prepare them for future contact with people with ASDs.

Suggestion Box

For younger children, diagrams can be used to present the triad of impairments as a strong but simple model. Younger pupils will benefit by hands-on experience of **PECS** (Picture Exchange Communication System) books and **TEACCH** (Treatment and Education of Autistic and related Communication handicapped CHildren) schedules and the use of video to observe how people with autism use these resources.

For older, able pupils, the shared reading of texts such as Mark Haddon's highly successful *The Curious Incident of the Dog in the Night-time*, Temple Grandin's *Emergence Labelled Autistic* or Donna Williams's *Nobody Nowhere* will provide the class with insights into the condition from an autistic perspective. Practitioners might choose to develop themes focused on literature from the field of autism.

Developing Understanding of Individual Needs

Given the breadth of the autistic spectrum, it will be necessary to develop the general shared information towards an understanding of the particular child with autism. This can be achieved by engaging the pupils in exercises which draw from them ideas about the difficulties faced by their classmate with autism. As indicated earlier this needs to be handled with great sensitivity and respect for the child with autism. Practitioners should be as objective as possible and avoid presenting the child as a curiosity.

> **Suggestion Box**
>
> Having taught the children about the general features of autism, present a lesson in which pupils are asked to:
>
> - Describe the difficulties their classmate encounters as a consequence of their autism.
>
> - Record the things that they know their classmate likes and the things they dislike.
>
> - List their classmate's strengths and qualities.
>
> - Suggest strategies which will support their classmate's learning.

Recognising Achievement

Time should be spent identifying the achievements of pupils with autism and enabling the children to understand that what may seem a small step for them, is a giant leap for their classmate with autism. By attaching value to the everyday achievements of the child a healthy message is shared by both the child with autism and their peers.

Deflating Peer Pressure

As we get older, most people desperately want to belong. Standing out is mortifying and those children who may previously have been happy to be seen as a companion for a child with an ASD may now seem to reject their friend in order to protect themself. Pre-empting this by encouraging friendship early in children's school careers may ensure that bonds are sufficiently strong to override this period. However, alone this is not enough; youngsters who are taking on the role of friend to a child with autism need to be supported through pastoral care and an explicit valuing of the role the youngster has adopted.

Appendix

Please photocopy the following materials, adapting as necessary to the context in which you are working and the nature of the group you are working with.

These resources are also available to download from the PCP website (www.paulchapmanpublishing.co.uk/resources/hanbury.pdf).

INSET Materials

Developing Practice for the Pupil with Autism

Aims:

1. Develop understanding of autism.
2. Consider learning needs based on this understanding.
3. Apply this knowledge to the working context.
4. Customise this knowledge to particular contexts.

Objective	Activity	Process	Resources	Time
To determine participants' existing understanding of autism.	Participants to write down what the term autism means to them. Colleagues then feedback description to whole group.	Have people complete this exercise individually, without discussion. You are after initial impressions, so only allow a minute or so for the description.	Pen, paper	15 minutes

Pause: Responses to this activity will provide you with an early impression of people's understanding. Time spent in discussing the definition presented in the next activity can be adjusted to meet the needs of the participants. It is important that an accurate and valid understanding of the condition is shared by all participants as early as possible in the training.

Objective	Activity	Process	Resources	Time
To provide a definition of autism based on established knowledge.	Trainer to provide definition of autism drawn from literature. Discuss the definition. Encourage people to relate this definition to the pupils they work with.	Use visual materials to show the definition.	OHT 1	15 minutes
To inform participants of current conceptual models of autism.	Trainer to review: • Triad of Impairments • Mind-blindness • Executive Function • Central Coherence Theory	Trainer to present models using visual materials. Provide written descriptions of each model for use in next activity.	OHTs 2–5	60 minutes

Pause: This has been a whistle stop tour of autism! Ensure that participants have references to further their knowledge if they wish to.

Educating Pupils with Autistic Spectrum Disorders © Martin Hanbury, 2005

Objective	Activity	Process	Resources	Time
To encourage participants to consider the impact of autism on a child's learning.	Group activity in which each group focuses on a model and lists how the features of that model will impact on a person's learning.	Form groups, give out descriptions of models. Group to list as many ways as they can think of in which the model impacts on learning. Follow by each group presenting this to the whole group. Discussion.	Flipcharts, markers	60 minutes
To enable participants to identify features of their current practice that might present obstacles to learning for a child with autism.	Individuals to reflect on their practice focusing on the obstacles to learning for a child with ASD in their classroom.	Have people complete this exercise individually, without discussion. Maintain this as a 'private' exercise.	Pen and paper	15 minutes
To inform participants of effective interventions for pupils with autism.	Trainer to review: • TEACCH • PECS	Trainer to present interventions using visual materials.	OHTs 6 and 7	60 minutes
To encourage participants to apply information in order to address the learning needs of pupils with autism.	Groups to devise realistic classroom scenarios identifying 3–5 obstacles to learning for pupils with ASDs. Groups to nominate strategies and means for implementing them in order to overcome these obstacles. Present for whole group discussion.	Form Groups. Provide support where necessary, offering concrete scenarios, providing concrete examples of difficulties. Allow ten minutes. Move group onto problem-solving section. Allow thirty minutes. Encourage in-depth discussion of each issue. Final plenary; each group to present.	Flipcharts, markers	60 minutes
To reflect on learning achieved.	Each member of the group to identify one issue that they will take away from the session.	Open discussion. Move round each group member. Encourage differing responses.		15 minutes

Educating Pupils with Autistic Spectrum Disorders © Martin Hanbury, 2005

What is Autism?

1. Autistic spectrum disorders is the term used to describe a range of behaviourally defined neurodevelopmental conditions.

2. They are characterised by impairments in:

   - social interaction

   - social communication and language development

   - a restricted repertoire of interests, behaviours and activities.

3. Sensory abnormalities and unusual interest in some sensations are common.

4. A lack of imaginative play indicates an underlying difficulty with generation of ideas that is highly relevant in the development of understanding other people and other situations.

5. All of these characteristics can be seen in varying degrees of severity.

6. As a developmental condition, the manifestation of autism for any one individual will vary:

   - across the lifespan

   - with maturation

   - according to the effects of different environments

   - due to specific interventions and treatments.

Source: Based on Charman, 2004: 4.

The Triad of Impairments

- social interaction

- social communication and

- imagination

'... we found that all children with "autistic features", whether they fitted Kanner's or Asperger's descriptions or had bits and pieces of both, had in common absence or impairments of social interaction, communication and development of imagination. They also had a narrow, rigid, repetitive pattern of activities and interests. The three impairments (referred to as the "triad") were shown in a wide variety of ways, but the underlying similarities were recognizable.'

Source: Wing, 1996: 25

Mind-blindness

- People with autism lack a 'theory of mind'.

- **Theory of Mind** is the ability to appreciate the mental states of oneself and other people.

- It is a prerequisite to effective functioning in social groups.

- It is usually evident in children from around the age of four upwards.

- However, children with autism seem to lack the ability to 'think about thoughts' (Happe, 1994).

Source: Based on Baron-Cohen, 1990, 1995 and Happe, 1994.

Executive Function

● This is the mechanism which enables us to move our attention from one activity or object to another flexibly and easily.

● It allows us to plan strategically, solve problems and set ourselves objectives.

● The absence of such a mechanism determines that:

1. all our actions are controlled by the environment in response to cues and stimuli, leading to apparently meaningless activity.

2. actions and behaviours compete for dominance in a disorganised and inconsistent manner leading to an inability to plan and execute goal-generated behaviour.

● In a school setting, this emerges as:

1. highly distractible behaviour

2. dependence upon ritual and routines

3. an apparent disregard for the school timetable or the completion of tasks.

Source: Based on Norman and Shallice, 1980.

Central Coherence Theory

- Natural impulse to place information into a context in order to give it meaning.

- People with autism tend to focus on the detail rather than the whole.

- The failure to appreciate the whole accounts for the piecemeal way in which people with autism acquire knowledge and the unusual cognitive profile presented by many people with autism.

- Educators may detect the lack of central coherence in:

  1. the narrowed interests of children with autism

  2. the ways in which pupils with autism are often unable to generalise skills

  3. the way in which children with autism often display areas of relative strength described as islets of ability.

Source: Based on Frith, 1989.

TEACCH

Treatment and **E**ducation of **A**utistic and related **C**ommunication handicapped **CH**ildren

● Lifelong programme for people with autism based on a recognition of characteristic strengths and typical impairments.

● Structured teaching has four major components:

1. physical organisation

2. schedules

3. work systems

4. task organisation.

● Structured teaching can be incorporated into mainstream practice through use of the four major components

Source: Based on Schopter and Mesibov, 1995 and Mesibov: 246–63, and Howley, 2003.

Educating Pupils with Autistic Spectrum Disorders © Martin Hanbury, 2005

PECS

Picture **E**xchange **C**ommunication **S**ystem

- Pictures provide permanence of information.

- Allow processing time which supports understanding.

- Learner initiates communicative acts.

- PECS takes the learner through six phases, namely:

  1. Phase One – Initiating Communication

  2. Phase Two – Expanding the Use of Pictures

  3. Phase Three – Choosing the Message in PECS

  4. Phase Four – Introducing the Sentence Structure in PECS

  5. Phase Five – Teaching Answering Simple Questions

  6. Phase Six – Teaching Commenting.

- Appropriate for pupils with language as it supports comprehension and allows extension of existing skills.

Source: Based on Bondy and Frost, 2002.

Chapter 4

Addressing Behavioural Issues in Autism

- Considers behavioural issues in terms of fear, flight and fight responses.

- Presents proven and effective strategies for addressing each level of response.

- Provides materials for planning behaviour support including flow chart for developing risk assessment and format for behaviour support plan.

Before we can begin to address the primary impact of autism we must develop strategies which are focused on the behavioural issues often associated with the condition. It is important to recognise that such behaviours are the result of the child's learning needs and are not themselves the learning need. Failure to appreciate this leads to the child's learning needs never being adequately addressed. However, these behavioural issues invariably present obstacles to the practitioner and therefore need to be minimised before we can get to the heart of the child's needs.

OVERCOMING FEAR

I am rationally aware that air travel is statistically far safer than any other form of transport. Nevertheless, I am scared of flying and such rationality counts for nothing when I arrive at the airport. Yet, I have developed a set of strategies to overcome my fear and so I board the plane, never happily, but I manage.

Compounded by autism, fear can appear impregnable. But it need not be and solutions lie in the same set of strategies which enable me to fly; in the same group of approaches which enable anybody to overcome their fears. These strategies need to be formed into a systematic and continuously evolving programme which is delivered consistently and skilfully across all aspects of the child's life. This systematic approach involves:

- accepting
- explaining
- desensitising
- supporting
- celebrating.

Accepting

There are two components to this element of the strategy. The first of these is to consider whether we do anything about the fear at all, whether what we gain for the child is worth the undoubted anxiety we will cause him/her. Consult widely with parents, colleagues, fellow professionals and practitioners before embarking upon a programme. Where appropriate, include the child in these discussions. Should we decide to implement a programme, the second component comes into play. This involves us deciding which aspects of the child's behaviour we are going to accept as necessary in enabling them to overcome fear. Many children with autism have intricate and precise rituals which may well be rooted in a 'fear response'. Indeed, most human beings, most human societies, use ritual to enable them to address potentially stressful situations. Therefore, as part of the programme, we must determine which of these rituals are indispensable to the child and which are detrimental to the child's overall development. We must also consider the affect of the child's 'ritualistic behaviour' on other children in the classroom. In mainstream settings a balance must be achieved between the needs of the child with autism and the needs of the whole group. It is often necessary to explain sensitively to the class group why certain things are acceptable for the child with autism whereas they are not for other children in the group.

CASE STUDY

Accepting

Alex returned from the summer vacation pretty much the way Alex had been before the break; happy, relaxed, making steady progress, comfortable with familiar people. That is, until the second Wednesday back. The taxi escort got bitten, the classroom staff were scratched and kicked. Alex cried bitterly all morning and as we set off for the swimming baths, the anxiety became palpable.

The following Wednesday Alex's mum called us before school. There had been a terrible scene at home and she was beside herself. Alex hadn't been like this for such a long time and mum had thought the bad times were over. She said, 'Do you think it's the swimming baths?' She was right. Whereas Alex had loved swimming previously, something had happened and now swimming was hell for Alex.

▶

For the rest of the term we tried everything we knew. There was lots of water-play in school, stories about going to the baths, paddling at the poolside, reward systems, low demands, no demands. We ran out of ideas. And still every Wednesday, Alex attacked anyone who came near and cried constantly until after lunch. One Wednesday, Alex's mum called before school and said, 'Can't we just forget it?' We agreed. The gain was not worth the pain, not for Alex. Alex was unlikely to ever use the swimming baths independently, enjoyed other forms of exercise and would happily engage in these, was in good general health and only noticeably distressed on Wednesday mornings. We decided to stop swimming lessons for Alex and Wednesday mornings immediately became calmer and more productive. Alex still does not swim.

Did we do the right thing?

Explaining

It is very important to let the child with autism know what is coming next in all arenas. When asking the child to confront their anxieties we are morally obliged to inform the child exactly what is being asked of them. Given the breadth of the spectrum, the means by which this information is passed is wide ranging. However, remember that everybody's ability to process information and express ideas diminishes considerably when they are in stressful situations. How eloquent are you when a car suddenly pulls out in front of you? Therefore, be prepared with a range of materials which support the explanations you are giving to children. Support the language you use with either written instructions or pictorial systems. Be sure to present the information in small, incremental units with a clear beginning, middle and end. Crucially, maintain whatever support system you have throughout the programme, constantly reiterating for the child what is happening. The child may be encouraged to adopt the sequence of events as a mantra which they repeat as they complete the given challenge.

CASE STUDY

Same Challenge, Different Child

This fear relates to entering the dining hall at lunch-time. In the first instance the child is an able, verbal youngster in a local primary school. In the second case, the child is a preverbal pupil in a generic Severe Learning Difficulties school. In both cases a visual system has been devised to explain the sequence of events to the child, one using words, the other using symbols.

Case One:

1 Walk down the corridor to the dining hall.
2 You will hear noises from the hall.
3 These noises are OK. It is the other children talking or moving about.

4   Go into the hall.

5   Stand in the line for your dinner.

6   Pick up a plate from the pile.

7   Choose the things you want to eat.

8   Take your plate to your place.

9   Eat your dinner.

10   When you have finished your dinner, take your plate to the hatch.

11   You may leave the dining hall and go to the library area.

12   The bell will ring at the end of break-time. You must go to class.

Case Two:

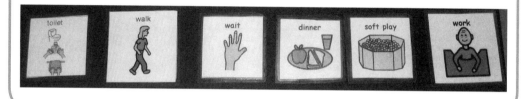

Desensitising

Desensitisation is a common component of any programme enabling a person to overcome their fears. In many ways, the term is something of a misnomer because we are not aiming to remove a child's sensitivities but rather to enable the child to cope with the sensations they experience in particular situations. At the heart of this process is familiarisation. The objective is to present the child with repeated positive experiences around the issue which has been causing them anxiety. However, difficulties arise in presenting situations which do not frighten the child further and yet remain relevant to the objective of the programme. There are several tools which can be used depending on the specific child and situation being addressed. These include:

- gradual introduction

- distraction techniques

- skilling up

- environmental familiarisation

- modelling, which may be used individually or as part of a combined programme of interventions.

Gradually introducing the child to the experience they find stressful may enable them to tolerate increasing exposure to the experience. This can be achieved across several dimensions:

1   An approach may be based around gradually increasing the amount of time a child can tolerate the experience.

2   Strategies may focus upon decreasing the physical distance a child is from the situation they find aversive.

3   An experience is broken into discrete components. The child is exposed to each of these individually and then collectively.

Suggestion Box

In this example the child is scared of school assemblies. Strategies from each of the three approaches discussed above are explored.

1   The child is only required to join the group for a set amount of time, for example, three minutes. After three minutes they can leave and go to their favourite place. Give the child a means of tracking time, such as a small sand timer or stopwatch. After several successful weeks at three minutes, increase the time to four, then five and so on.

2   The child sits in the corridor outside the hall. Over time, gradually move the place they sit closer to the hall door. Eventually move the place into the main hall.

3   Video a school assembly. Show the child the video over several sessions, watching a minute or two at a time. Meanwhile, take the child into the main hall when it is empty. Get them to sit on a chair in a fixed place which they are comfortable with. Expose the child to small sections of recorded applause. Gradually bring each of these components together.

Apply the principles behind these strategies to the particular area of fear you are addressing. Judging the pace at which each new element is introduced is the real test of the practitioner's skill.

Distraction techniques have served parents throughout the ages and continue to be an enduring and effective way of diverting a child's attention away from the object of fear. Whilst these techniques are particularly useful in addressing one-off difficulties, such as injections or sudden thunderstorms, they have limited value when concerned with regular experiences which are part of the child's everyday life. Such experiences need to be addressed rather than circumvented and distraction techniques tend to hide issues as opposed to enabling a child to overcome them.

Suggestion Box

Always have a handy supply of things that help the child cope. Favourite toys, familiar songs or music, set conversations on favourite topics are all invaluable in one-off stressful situations. The use of these props should be temporary; it is far better to work towards enabling the child to overcome their fear.

Skilling up involves teaching the child the skills they will need to overcome their fear away from the context which they associate with the fear. For example, a child who becomes scared of going into the playground because of difficulties with peers might be taught to cope with these pressures through role play or social stories. Equipped with these skills the child must then be taught to transfer these strategies to the original scenario.

Environmental familiarisation is a useful approach for children who may have an aversion to a particular feature which can be introduced gradually into a context in which a child is known to be secure and happy. A common use of this technique is in relation to sounds which pupils find aversive. These can be recorded and played very softly to the child whilst the child is in a place which feels safe to them. Gradually the volume or duration of these sounds can be increased until the child is confident when faced with this sound in its original context.

Modelling is effective where children have either particular trust of a person or a tendency to copy behaviour. It is possible to use either feature to enable the child to learn through modelling a strategy which will allow them to overcome the barrier created by their fear.

CASE STUDY

Imran

Imran didn't like swimming. But he did like Mandy. So when it came to swimming sessions, Mandy would hold his hand and stroll casually along the side of the pool, singing softly to herself. After a couple of weeks of doing this, she started to dip her foot into the water every so often. The following week she knelt down and splashed her hands in the water. Imran started to copy.

The next week Mandy sat on the side dangling her feet in the pool and within a few weeks she had climbed waist-deep into the water. Imran had followed her and was soon taking the lead, becoming more and more adventurous with each passing week until he began to splash about on his own.

Supporting

This component of the programme has many and varied facets. For some pupils support might be overt and explicit, involving many members of staff and considerable resources. For other pupils it may be subtle, infrequent or casual, yet just as effective for the intended purpose. Support can come in the form of encouragement, persistence, advocacy, resources, supporting supporters, counselling and a host of other incarnations. However, despite this range of means and methods there are certain universal qualities which must be present for support to be effective. The first of these is that support must be thoroughly planned and tailored to the unique needs of the child. Secondly, support must be consistent and reliable and not prone to sudden, disastrous withdrawal. Finally, support must be expert, delivered by knowledgeable people with sufficient experience and continuous training.

A Spectrum of Support The most cognitively able child with autism can experience the severest disability as a consequence of the condition. The impact of autism may not be obvious in the academic security of the classroom but may become achingly apparent during unstructured break-times or when completing open-ended tasks. Support for this child needs to be targeted at those times when the condition's impact is at its greatest.

Other children with autism can be both severely disabled cognitively and severely impaired across the triad. These children require intensive support throughout their lives, often involving many agencies. A high level of expertise is necessary to meet the needs of these children and managers of services need to ensure sufficient support and training is available to practitioners.

Celebrating

There is a myth that children with ASDs neither care about praise nor respond to positive language. It is my experience celebrating the success of a child with an ASD is just as important and just as productive as it is for any child. Furthermore, overcoming fear for any person is a major achievement; for a child with autism it is the pinnacle of endeavour. Consequently, celebrating the child's success must be an integral part of any programme targeted at overcoming their fear response. The nature of this celebration will vary according to the needs and strengths of each individual, but must be based on those things that the child finds rewarding and satisfying. A well chosen celebration of the child's achievement will reinforce the success and lead to further achievements in an ever broadening experience of the world.

FLIGHT RESPONSES

Flight can take many forms ranging from the child physically running away from situations to the child who dominates conversations in order to avoid directed tasks and activities. However, at the heart of each form of this behaviour is the core desire to escape the situation in which the child finds him/herself. Strategies may vary, but the recognition that this type of behaviour fulfils a fundamental need for the child must inform any approach which is adopted. Approaches that only deal with the behaviour we see, will be short-term and superficial in their effect. Real progress lies in removing the need for the child to escape, that is, in addressing the root cause of the behaviour. This is often very difficult because the original cause of the behaviour has disappeared under the rubble of time and can no longer be detected. The original cause can transform, so that, whereas the child originally escaped because something in the room distressed them or something outside the room attracted them, the child now runs away because it is fun and stimulating to do so. Consequently, addressing the root cause of the behaviour is an exercise in archaeology, gradually peeling away layers in order understand the motives and needs of the child. This detective work involves broad consultation of people in the child's life, close examination of any notes or records and targeted observations of the child in a variety of contexts. It can be lengthy and sometimes fruitless work which must be conducted with great sensitivity to both the child and other people involved with the child. It is crucial to avoid suggestions of blame or encourage unfounded speculations which may harden into unhelpful opinions.

Running Away

Of the various forms of flight, this is potentially the most dangerous and presents the most immediate challenge to practitioners. Children with autism are often impulsive and usually have a very poor awareness of danger, resulting in a high risk of harm to themselves or to those attempting to rescue them. Prevention is infinitely better than cure and a thorough risk assessment is an indispensable component of practice with any child with ASDs. Always assume a worst case scenario and remember that pupils with autism can be incredibly resourceful and alert to opportunities for escape. As we know, the best laid plans can fail and there needs to be well rehearsed contingency arrangements. Ask yourself at each stage of escape – be it out of the work area, out of the classroom or out of the school – *what will happen if …?*

The following flow chart (Figure 4.1) is intended to suggest a process for developing risk assessment. Please note, the flow chart is not a risk assessment; these should be developed within the context in which you are working as each situation is unique. Risk assessment must be a dynamic process, informed by observation and analysis and responsive to changes. A risk assessment may be documented, but it is never completed.

Figure 4.1   Flow chart for Risk Assessment

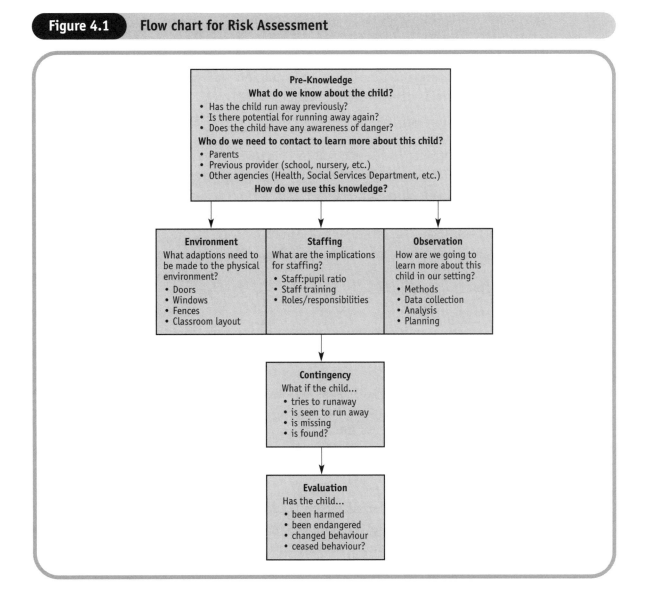

Refusal

Refusing to engage in or complete activities can be the hardest form of behaviour for many practitioners to understand. We might well feel that we have done everything we can to make the activity accessible for the child, have judged that the child should be able to achieve success in the task, have planned scrupulously for all eventualities and yet, the child refuses to engage. Refusal appears obstinate and undermines our perception of ourselves as professionals, creating negative feelings and profound frustration. However, this form of behaviour requires as much analysis and proactive planning as those behavioural types which might win our sympathy more readily because it is rooted in those same areas of impairments which cause difficulties for the learner with autism.

Approaches towards the child's refusal to work must begin with the practitioner adjusting their mindset to a neutral setting, to the practitioner 'driving in neutral'. In order to achieve this, try to:

- avoid being drawn into a power struggle with the child

- focus on your objective and not the personalities involved

- take the demands of time out of the situation – completing the task tomorrow is as valuable as completing it today

- act as a broker between the child and the task – don't become the task.

Once the practitioner has separated the needs of the child from the demands of the situation, a thorough process of investigation into what it is about the task that is causing difficulties can begin. Break down the task into its elemental parts; include in this analysis each resource used, every part of the working environment and the teaching strategies adopted as well as the basic content of the lesson itself. Difficulties may arise from a minor component of the lesson which has immense significance for the child with autism; it may be something that we could easily replace or substitute with another element.

Give particular attention to the amount of processing time the child has for each element of the lesson. Much of our success or failure in teaching children with autism lies in our ability to pace lessons properly. Often refusal is caused by a child not comprehending fully what is required of them. Remember for a person with autism not understanding fully is not understanding at all. Also remember that a child who can process information very quickly in one area, may be very poor at processing information in other areas and that the capacity to process information will vary from day to day and environment to environment.

Consider the support materials which could be used to enable the child to complete the task. Regardless of the child's cognitive ability, the presented task may appear overwhelming to them. Provide the child with lists of instructions, pictorial cues or a model of the end product. For many children with autism, the process of handwriting can be very difficult and painful; allow the use of computers wherever necessary. Should anybody oppose your use of supportive materials, claiming an unfair advantage to the child, remind them that as with any prosthetic, where there is a need, there should be a system of support.

> ### Suggestion Box
>
> Providing a model of 'closed tasks', such as numeracy problems or scientific experiments, is comparatively straightforward. Just give an example of how a problem should be presented or how an experiment might be reported.
>
> 'Open tasks', such as creative writing or artwork, present more difficulty. Provide four or five key instructions for the task, for example:
>
> 1 the story must contain five characters
> 2 the story must take place in three different places
> 3 there must be a secret in the story
> 4 the story must end in a strange house.

Obsession

This aspect of the flight response is itself a defining feature of autism (Kanner, 1943). In developing strategies to address this area we must give consideration to the reasons the child is engaged in this type of behaviour. If it is to structure a confusing, muddled world, then we must apply approaches which enable the child to structure their understanding. If it is to block out unpleasant sensations, then we must either find the means to increase the child's tolerance of these sensations or remove the sensations altogether. If it is to engage in pleasurable sensations, then we must find ways of replicating these sensations via a broader range of experiences. We must also give thought as to whether we interfere at all.

Whilst obsession is a complex area to address, there are strategies and approaches which can be employed to engage a child. These rely on our skills as practitioners to interest and motivate the learner, remembering that what interests the child with autism may not be readily apparent to us. Therefore, we need to take the time to observe the child, learn what it is that motivates them and, more challengingly, learn what it is about what it is that motivates them, that motivates them. Having, discovered this, we need to become skilled in the experience that the child finds interesting so that we become an important resource to the child, someone who is interesting. From here we can then adapt activities to engage the child using ourselves as a conduit to the task. Become expert in the child's field of interest, whether it be the skill of spinning small toys or the dynasties of Ancient Egypt; become important to the child.

UNDERSTANDING VIOLENT BEHAVIOUR

Sadly, for some people with autism it is only when they resort to violence that their needs are met. This violence may be directed towards others, towards themselves or towards property. This behaviour, which is highly effective, becomes ingrained and, therefore, difficult to replace with more appropriate means of meeting needs. Often, resources are driven by crises rather than preventative intervention, resulting in a demoralising cycle of events in which early indicators are ignored, preventative opportunities are missed and violent behaviour escalates. Consequently, resources are diverted from good preventative practice towards expensive, often ineffective, crisis management. Courage and foresight are needed amongst commissioners of services in order to end this cycle and focus on the quality of life of the individuals the service is serving.

The key to this is early intervention. Inevitably, the younger the child concerned, the more likely a positive outcome. Paradoxically, it is sometimes harder to detect early warning signs with younger children as potentially violent behaviour is often dismissed as tantrums the child will grow out of. Unfortunately, for the child with a limited repertoire of skills, the chances of growing out of the behaviour, particularly if it is extremely effective, are reduced. It is therefore crucial to teach the child, as early as possible, alternatives to this behaviour. Since the impact of a young child's violence is comparatively light, because the behaviour can be contained and ignored, there is the tendency for people to disregard the behaviour and fail to act. However, the continuation of this behaviour is extremely damaging for the child and the skilled intervention of adults is of paramount importance. Intervention should focus on:

- identification

- needs

- alternatives

- consistency.

The accurate and precise identification of the behaviour is a crucial first step. Try and be as specific as possible, avoid general comments and focus on the particular behaviour which is causing difficulty. Attempt to identify the context in which the behaviour occurs and try to quantify how often and for how long the behaviour is evident. It is as important to analyse when behaviour is not occurring as it is to identify when it is. Use this period of identification to dispel any myths which may have accumulated. Common phrases, such as 'he does it all the time' or 'this happens every time,' need to be weighed against the facts.

Challenging behaviour is driven by needs. The more limited a person's options for meeting their needs, the more likely they are to develop behaviour which is challenging. Whenever we encounter challenging behaviour, the first question we must ask ourselves is, 'What need is this behaviour meeting?' Invariably, the answer to the question is a very basic need such as discomfort, stimulus, hunger, thirst, fear or loneliness. The one thing we can be certain of is that we cannot drive away the need. We can alter the behaviour which we see but we cannot change the need. We must address the need either by our own actions or by teaching the child to address the need themselves.

If we can accurately identify the need driving the behaviour, we have the opportunity to address and reduce the behaviour. The following Needs Checklist can be used to determine the driving force behind the child's behaviour. This can be used in this form or adapted to meet the specific circumstances the practitioner is working in.

Needs Checklist

When .... exhibits this behaviour is he/she

1. hungry

2. thirsty

3. frightened

4. in pain

5. uncomfortable

6. bored

7. lonely

8. over-stimulated

9. desperate for the toilet

10. anxious

11. missing somebody

12. angry

13. excited

14. sexually aroused

15. insecure

Often practitioners find that there are several needs operating simultaneously. This presents practitioners with a significant dilemma. Whilst it is true that aiming to do everything usually results in achieving nothing, we must also consider that in the field of challenging behaviour, the complex and shifting interplay of needs dictates that we must address several dimensions of need at the same time. There are various ways this can be done. For example, having identified the needs frightened, uncomfortable, over-stimulated, angry and insecure using the checklist, practitioners may grade (Figure 4.2) each component according to its influence on the behaviour. Practitioners can then decide whether they wish to:

1   focus entirely on the need with the most profound influence (Figure 4.3)

2   address a hierarchy of needs, such as the three most influential (Figure 4.4)

3   focus attention on an area of need in proportion to its influence (Figure 4.5)

This approach can be represented as follows

Figure 4.2   Grading Needs

Grade needs 1–10 where the highest scores reflect the most profound influence on behaviour.

frightened	4
uncomfortable	5
over-stimulated	8
angry	2
insecure	1

Figure 4.3   Priority

Focusing solely on the dominant issue.

over-stimulated	8

Figure 4.4 Hierachy

Concentrating on the three most influential areas.

over-stimulated	8
uncomforatble	5
frightened	4

Figure 4.5 Proportion

Add up the values for each need. Calculate the pertcentage of the total represented by each figure. Dedicate that proportion of your efforts towards addressing that specific need.

Need	Grade	Percentage
frightened	4	20
uncomfortable	5	25
over-stimulated	8	40
angry	2	10
insecure	1	5
Total 20		100

It is essential to remember that we cannot take away the need. Our work should focus on providing the child with alternatives to the behaviour in order to meet the needs. Alternatives must be successful and reliable if the child is to adopt them. They must be powerful reinforcers of positive behaviour and often require us to adapt our practice in order to consistently and reliably reward positive responses.

It is useful to think of several phases of alternatives. The first phase must be easily accessible to the child, have an immediate effect and provide the child with many opportunities for easy success. These early successes can provide a platform for alternatives which require the child to use newly acquired skills such as enhanced communication strategies or anger management strategies.

From this progress, alternatives can focus upon delaying the reward for positive behaviour further still via the use of token systems or the celebration of good work. The two case studies, Alternatives for Kelly and Alternatives for Josh, show broad examples intended only to illustrate key principles.

Alternatives for Kelly

Kelly attacks members of staff in response to demand for work. This is generally understood as an attempt to avoid the work task.

Objective 1 – Provide Kelly with an alternative way of avoiding tasks.

- Strategy 1 – Teach Kelly to give a 'break' symbol to the member of staff whenever she wants to avoid work tasks. Each time Kelly attempts to hit you, block the attempt and hold up the break symbol. Encourage Kelly to begin using this symbol to obtain a break.
- Outcome 1 – This will result in Kelly using the break symbol each time she wants to opt out. Initially, this will be acceptable because the symbol has to work.

Objective 2 – Enable Kelly to tolerate longer periods of time before a break is given.

- Strategy 2 – Teach Kelly to wait ten seconds after giving the break symbol before she takes a break. When she gives you the symbol begin counting. Gradually build up the number of seconds you are counting for.
- Outcome 2 – Kelly will learn to delay the period of time between a behaviour and its desired effect.

Objective 3 – Teach Kelly to work for sustained periods of time following a routine which incorporates a break at an allotted time.

- Strategy 3 – Present Kelly with a work schedule which shows the break symbol. Talk Kelly through a sequence of 'work first, then break.'
- Outcome 3 – Kelly will learn to rely on the prospect of the break coming and will tolerate increasing periods of demand.

Alternatives for Josh

Josh bites other children during unstructured play-times. It is generally understood that this is done to gain adult attention.

Objective 1 – Provide Josh with an alternative way of gaining adult attention.

- Strategy 1 – Identified adult will focus on Josh throughout play-time, directing him into activities and engaging him in one-to-one play if Josh becomes agitated. Josh is frequently praised (three times per minute) for positive behaviour.
- Outcome 1 – Other children are protected from attacks by Josh. Josh will become dependent upon the adult's attention during play-times.

Objective 2 – Enable Josh to cope without adult attention for short periods of time.

- **Strategy 2** – Encourage Josh to play independently for up to one minute. Every minute praise Josh and show him you have put a tick on his 'tick chart'. At the end of the session, encourage Josh to count how many ticks he has gained.
- **Outcome 2** – Josh will learn the value of positive adult attention. His dependency will be gradually reduced.

Objective 3 – Josh will play independently for up to five minutes.

- **Strategy 3** – Josh will be taught to come and tell an identified person that he has played nicely every five minutes. Use a sand timer to inform Josh of the time.
- **Outcome 3** – Josh will learn to monitor his own behaviour and judge acceptable behaviour.

Having identified the behaviour, isolated the need driving the behaviour and provided the child with alternative means of addressing that need, it is vital that we achieve consistency across all settings in order to support the child. Consistent approaches rely upon consensus between all significant parties in the child's life with regard to the way a particular behaviour is addressed. If this is not achieved, it is unrealistic to expect everyone involved to adhere to the proposed strategy. If approaches are not consistent, it is unlikely that the child's learning will be generalised and, therefore, become firmly embedded. Consequently, when planning behaviour support for a child, it is crucial to involve everyone with significant input into the child's life.

It is advisable to design a written behaviour support programme in order to enable a close focus on the target behaviour and consistent approaches towards it. Plans should focus on providing alternatives to challenging behaviour through proactive programmes, which teach skills relevant to the needs of the child. The plan should also include active strategies, which can be used if the child is becoming anxious or distressed and help to diffuse or distract the child. If the child enters into challenging behaviour a series of planned and predictable responses or reactive strategies should be employed. Across all three dimensions consistency is essential. We cannot expect the child to progress if we cannot guarantee our responses and share our expectations.

Behaviour Support Plan

Name:	Class:	Programme:	Date:	Review:

Behaviour:

Need:

Objective:

Proactive Strategies	Active Strategies	Reactive Strategies

Written by:	Consulted:	Agreed by:

Despite our best efforts to prevent violent behaviour before it becomes deeply ingrained, we may meet pupils for whom this behaviour has been an effective and functional form for a prolonged period of time. It is essential that colleagues in such situations are given opportunities for accredited training in the area of behaviour support. Children with this degree of difficulty are highly complex and organisations catering for such children have a duty of care toward their staff and should ensure they are adequately equipped by specialists in the field to deal with such challenges. A number of established schemes are available and are best accessed via **BILD** (British Institute of Learning Disabilities).

Chapter 5

Understanding the Affect of the Condition

- Presents strategies to develop the child's understanding of the social context of the classroom.

- Suggests approaches to support effective communication.

- Discusses ways in which flexible thinking, problem solving and independence can be promoted.

The core deficits of autism are often obscured by a myriad of different factors. All too often, strategies are directed at other levels of impact of the condition without addressing the core impairments. Consequently, children do not make the progress they are capable of and become caught in an unproductive cycle of narrow learning and low expectation. For children with autism to progress well, approaches must address the fundamental impairments of autism and develop practice which is specific to condition.

SOCIAL UNDERSTANDING IN THE CLASSROOM

How can we support the child with autism in making sense of the blurring non-sense of the classroom? Firstly, we must identify those features of classroom society which are intolerable for the pupil with autism, including:

- unpredictability

- sensory overload

- interpreting emotions

- processing time.

Some children with autism will be able to learn how to overcome some of these features via a remedial curriculum; other children may need to develop skills which compensate for their inability to cope with the challenge (Jordan and Powell, 1995: 69–70). For example, one child may be taught to cope with a primary school assembly by gradual, carefully monitored introductions to larger and larger groups; another child may be taught a socially acceptable means of leaving the assembly when it becomes difficult for them to cope. In the first case the child's difficulties have been remedied whereas in the other, they have been compensated for. Whatever approach is adopted, a range of strategies need to be developed for each area of difficulty for the child.

Unpredictability

This has two distinct but related dimensions, namely the unpredictability of people and the unpredictability of events. The first of these is the hardest to legislate for; human beings are strange, unpredictable animals. Yet, we can introduce controls to the classroom situation which make the behaviour of other people easier for children with ASDs to predict. This should begin with you, the practitioner, working with the child. Develop your practice so that as many details as possible are regular, habitual and predictable. You may need to consider facets as diverse as the clothing you wear, the materials you use with the child or the names by which you address colleagues. Having ensured that your personal practice is predictable, develop consistent approaches with all colleagues. Start with those people who are in regular, direct contact with the child and spread this consistency to all members of staff. By designing a pupil profile it is possible to share, in an immediately accessible format, the things which colleagues need to know about a child; this will help promote consistency across the staff team.

Whilst enabling colleagues to be consistent should be relatively straightforward, encouraging the child's peers to be similarly predictable is problematic especially within a mainstream setting where practitioners will often actively encourage spontaneity and the use of initiative. It may be possible to discuss with the child's peers the need to behave in a way which is helpful to the child with autism; a discussion that can be based on previous work, raising the group's awareness of the condition. In other situations this may not be so easy due to the difficulties the peer group experience or, indeed, share with the child. In these circumstances, the onus falls upon our day-to-day practice to provide security and assurance to each child in the group, thereby encouraging predictable behaviour.

Pupil Profile

Name:	DOB:	Class:	Year:	Term:

Contacts:

Communication:

Self-help skills:

Known risks:

Dietary issues:

Medical information:

Likes	Dislikes:

Structuring the day so that a predictable, reliable routine is established is at the heart of all good practice for pupils with autism. We know that people with autism have difficulties in organising their ideas and in perceiving order around them. Consequently, a routine becomes an absolute necessity, a prerequisite for achievement. Communicating this routine is as important as the routine itself; having a routine is no good if the child with autism doesn't know about it! The seminal work of Division TEACCH, founded in North Carolina in the late 1960s, is based on these principles of establishing a routine and communicating it effectively to the child. Further study or training in this area is highly recommended. In the meantime, ensure that your practice in the following key areas is consistent and predictable.

Language and communication are crucial. Use set phrases or symbols for crucial components of the day or for activities the child finds difficult. Use a minimal amount of language when addressing potentially difficult times, remembering that the child's processing skills may be significantly diminished at these points.

Transitions are invariably a stressful time for children with autism and they need to be managed carefully and with skill. Give warnings of transitions and try to ensure that regular transitions, such as coming into school, going to dinner or using the toilet, happen at a set time and in a set pattern.

Establish a Daily Routine and ensure that you communicate it effectively to the child. This can be done in writing or by using symbols or pictures. The use of a schedule (Mesibov, 2003) for children with autism would be regarded as good practice; the length of the schedule will vary according to the child's ability to project forwards in time. Define the day for the child through a series of predictable markers or milestones, that is, activities which always occur at the same time, in the same place, in the same way.

Suggestion Box

1 The start of the school day is of vital importance for children with autism. Devise an individual morning routine based on the needs of the child. For some children, a very low demand, minimally interactive start to the day is necessary; for others, adult directed activities and a high degree of adult attention is preferred.

2 Following the individual routine, Greeting Time can be used to draw the child into the group using photographs to explain who is in school. Use symbols or words to describe what is expected during the day and music to focus the child on the information being shared.

3 Music is a fantastic resource for practitioners working with pupils with ASDs. Music is both structured and sensory, hence its power for pupils with autism. Use music to start and finish activities. You may do this by playing calming music at the beginning and end of activities or you may sing songs which are familiar cues to the child.

● Sensory Overload

People with autism are susceptible to sensory overload inducing states of either high excitability or high anxiety. The mechanisms involved in producing these responses are complex and rooted in the causes of autism detailed in Chapter 1. As practitioners, we are obliged to develop learning environments from the perspective of the child with autism. Jordan and Powell (1995) refer to an environment being 'optimally stimulating' and this term should be at the forefront of our thinking as we endeavour to create a bespoke classroom for the child.

Where colleagues are operating in autism specific environments, this is more straightforward than it is for those in situations where the child with autism is sharing a classroom with mainstream peers. In either circumstance, the starting point must be an analysis of the child's needs set within the context in which you are operating. Some adaptations may be relatively straightforward, others might be wholesale and inevitably costly. Whatever situation you are in, ensuring that the classroom has been appropriately designed around the child's sensory needs is vital. If we cannot achieve a learning environment which decreases the effect of sensory overload, the child is not going to be in a position to learn consistently and enduringly.

Practitioners are trained to develop exciting and stimulating classrooms and it is in their nature to immerse themselves in the creation of these environments. However, we need to ask ourselves: 'Is this right for the child we are working with?'; 'How does he/she see this?'; 'What does he/she hear, smell, feel or taste in the world created for him/her?'

The Sensory Overload Checklist may help in the development of your learning environment. In completing this checklist, it is crucial to consider the perspective of the child on which you are focusing. His or her needs will be unique and you must get as close as you can to how the child perceives the world.

In the columns Sensory Issue and Sense, identify the difficulty you feel the child faces and the sense you feel this relates to. For example, the following plan has been designed for Dan, an eight-year-old boy, who attends his local primary school, supported by an assistant. For Dan, you may write:

Sensory Issue	Sense
The sound of children's chairs scraping on the floor when they stand up to go out to play	Auditory

Sensory Overload Checklist

Sensory Issue	Sense	A	E	Feature of Context	Minimise Impact	Resolve

A = aversive
E = exciting

It is important to specify the issue you are targeting rather than provide vague, generalised statements. Furthermore, by isolating the sense you believe to be at the centre of the issue, you will gradually build up a documented pattern of need which may be helpful in the future.

It is then important to record whether the child finds this sensation aversive or exciting. This may change over time, and a record will be invaluable if the issue surfaces again. The next column, Feature of Context, places the issue within the real, practical situation in which you are working. Teaching is the art of the possible and this aspect of the checklist encourages the practitioner to focus their thinking on the reality they experience. Within the example given, this column might read:

Feature of Context
There are 31 children in the class; playtime is at 10:30 a.m.; all the children stand behind their chairs before going out to play; the first table ready are the first to go, so the children rush to be ready first

The final two columns are bred of pragmatism. The first of these considers strategies, which can be adopted in order to minimise the problem, whilst longer term resolutions are sought. For children with autism, doing nothing is rarely an option. Therefore, it is recommended that interim measures are taken in order to lessen the impact of sensory overload at the same time as looking for a more enduring solution. These columns might appear as follows:

Minimise Impact	Resolve
Dan leaves room three minutes before other children	Dan will be gradually desensitised to scraping noise
Class rewarded for getting ready quietly – particular attention to scraping of chairs	Classroom carpeted

It is likely that there will be several issues to be considered and these can be contained in the same plan, providing an overview of the child's needs profile. Dan's might look something like this:

Dan's Sensory Overload Checklist

Sensory Issue	Sense	A	E	Feature of Context	Minimise Impact	Resolve
The sound of children's chairs scraping on the floor when they stand up to go out and play	Auditory	*		There are 31 children in the class; playtime is at 10:30 a.m.; all the children stand behind their chairs before going out to play; the first table ready are the first to go, so the children rush to be ready first	Dan leaves room three minutes before other children Class rewarded for getting ready quietly – particular attention to scraping of chairs	Dan will be gradually desensitised to scraping noise Classroom carpeted
Car alarms in staff car park	Auditory		*	Dan's current classroom ajoins the staff car park Several members of staff have very sensitive alarms	Encourage colleagues to rectify alarms Dan to leave the room when alarms go off ostensibly to inform staff member alarm has gone off	Dan to have opportunities to listen to car alarms as a structured activity Future classroom away from car park

Interpreting emotions

Learning is an emotional exercise. Pupils and practitioners share joy, frustration, excitement or disappointment as they strive to extend their knowledge and skills. This sharing of emotion strengthens the bond between pupil and practitioner and thereby strengthens practice. Where a child has difficulty:

- recognising

- understanding or

- expressing

emotional states, this bond can be impaired. Therefore, a significant amount of time should be devoted to addressing this difficulty. Naturally, a child's cognitive ability has an influence on the extent to which progress can made in this area. However, the benefits of activities related to emotional development are significant and profound for all children regardless of their cognitive ability and approaches towards this end must therefore be pursued. As indicated above there are three chief components to this area of developmental need, each of which merits separate consideration.

Recognition. For the child with autism, this involves recognising emotions in both themselves and in other people. Once again the use of visual materials can be an effective approach for either element. Whilst, the child's cognitive ability and level of maturity will determine the materials used, a general process of working from the self outwards, that is, recognising their own emotions before recognising those emotions in others, is generally more effective. Initially, the pupil might focus on a narrow range of polar opposites, such as 'happy and sad', or 'like and dislike', applying these to themselves in familiar situations. From here, the range of emotions may be expanded before the child learns to interpret the emotional state of others from their facial expressions or actions. A more sophisticated range of activities might focus on inferring emotional states from contextual cues, such as 'Jack cannot find his coat' or 'Emma's Mummy is poorly.' Work in this area can be supported by resources including an excellent software program called 'Mindreading' by Simon Baron-Cohen.

Understanding. Understanding emotion requires a sophisticated matrix of skills which, for children with ASDs, presents many difficulties. In the context of working with children with autism, understanding emotion might be restricted to enabling the child to understand the likely causes, and probable outcomes, of an emotional state. Whilst limited, such an approach focuses on logical conclusions rather than requiring the pupil to engage aspects of their comprehension which are impaired. Initially, work may focus on the *cause* of emotional states and be based in the child's immediate experiences; 'Gareth is happy because it is his birthday.' As understanding develops here, learning can progress towards appreciating the *effect* of emotional states and be based at a greater emotional distance; 'Susie was sad and did not want to talk to her friends.' Should the child show a greater degree of empathic awareness, then a more expansive programme of work can be developed, moving the child away from concrete examples and simple emotional states towards dilemmas and situations outside the child's immediate experience.

Expression. There are several components to this area of difficulty for children with autism. There are children who can be inexpressive, who show little or no emotional response when it might be expected that other people would. There are youngsters who can be inappropriately expressive, who perhaps laugh when upset or in unfortunate situations, such as at funerals. Some children with autism are excessively expressive in that they seem to overreact to emotional stimuli, laughing loudly at moderately funny things or crying profusely when mildly upset. Some children are unpredictably expressive in that at times their emotional responses seem entirely appropriate, whereas at others, their responses are inexplicable.

Our aim as practitioners is to develop not only the child's repertoire of expression but also to enable them to monitor their responses. Again the breadth of the spectrum necessitates the use of a range of strategies. For some children, the use of symbols is most appropriate, encouraging the child to express their feelings in broad, simple terms. For other children, a phrase book of appropriate expressions for set situations might enable the child to comment upon their emotional state serving not only the child's needs but also our efforts to support those needs. For other children, social stories, presented either as written narratives (Gray, 1994a) or comic strips (Gray, 1994b), can provide scenarios which develop the child's understanding of appropriate modes and means of expression. This can establish a virtuous spiral wherein the child learns to manage social situations more effectively, gaining broader experience of social situations, thereby further developing their social skills.

Processing time

People with autism appear to process the information they receive from the world around them in a significantly different way to other people. It is not helpful to think of this difference *quantitatively*, that is in terms of thinking slower or faster than others, or having a greater or lesser capacity for learning, because the learning profiles of people with autism are characteristically unorthodox and uneven. It is more helpful to think of this difference in *qualitative* terms; in terms of the way people with autism think and the nature of their ability to process information. A useful metaphor for this is to visualise thought processes as a shape. Whereas most people's processing can be envisaged as a regular shape (a square, a triangle, a circle), for people with autism, irregular or abstract forms better describe the way in which their thought processes operate. In the classroom environment this presents significant problems for both the learner and the practitioner. For the child in specialist provision, these difficulties can be minimised as we learn more about the shape of their thinking and adapt the curriculum, activities and materials around them to suit their way of thinking. For the child in a mainstream classroom, the challenge is to alter a curriculum, which is exclusively based on regular shapes for the conventional learner, and a practice, which is developed for the majority.

In either context, the skilled practitioner employs approaches which recognise the difference in processing strategies that characterise the child with autism. Practitioners need to incorporate the following features in order to support the child's processing of information:

- time

- guidance

- relevant points

- small steps

- supportive materials

- silence

- refocusing strategies.

Children with autism need time to absorb information and prepare a response. This aspect of their learning is not related to the child's cognitive ability, so we cannot make assumptions that the more able the child the quicker the process. People with autism do not tend to see the big picture and need time in order to piece the bits of information they have into a coherent whole. In addition to this, many people with autism have difficulty in retrieving information. As a result, each time a child with autism is presented with a task, it may appear to the child that it is the first time that they have encountered this challenge. Consequently, even familiar tasks have to be relearned many times before they can become embedded in the child's repertoire of skills.

Children with autism will not instinctively orientate to the important information related to a task. Guidance can be provided in many ways depending upon the child's ability, the demands of the task and the learning context. For more able pupils, highlighter pens can be used to draw their attention to salient information. For children with a greater degree of learning difficulty, it is advisable to present only the necessary materials and information in order to complete the task.

Related to this feature is the need to focus the child's attention on the relevant points in a task. It is important to cut out any 'background noise' which may distract the child and cause them to deviate from the task. For example, many worksheets and textbooks, which are effective with pupils, contain illustrations designed to entertain the child. A child with autism can find these extremely distracting and fixate upon a component of the presentation which has little to do with the task itself. Practitioners may need to adapt these materials in order to meet the needs of the child with autism. Other children, involved in elementary tasks may find the actual materials themselves distracting and fixate upon the sensory features of the equipment. In these circumstances it is necessary to consider how you might maintain the learning content of the task using different, 'neutral' materials.

In order to prevent the child becoming overwhelmed by the task, it is important to present the task as a series of small steps, each with a distinct beginning and ending. This will ensure that the child meets with success at frequent milestones along the way, encouraging them in the task and building confidence and self-esteem. For example, an able child with autism working on a series of numeracy problems might record each time he has completed a problem on a tally chart. A less able youngster, might receive a small reward each time a component of a relatively complex task is completed.

Supportive materials including written lists, symbols and pictures, which focus the child on the task and constantly remind the child what is required of them, are invaluable for many children with autism. Where possible present the child with a representation of the end product in order to enable them to understand what they are working towards and what it will look like when it is finished. Sometimes, the best support material available is the practitioner themself.

It is important for practitioners to develop their practice to allow opportunities for the child to respond. For children with autism silence can be golden. However, as practitioners we often verbally encourage, rephrase questions or offer helpful prompts if a child is apparently struggling to respond. This persistent encouragement could be seen as oppressive to children with autism and may add to the difficulty they are experiencing in focusing on the task. Practitioners need to make a conscious effort to leave gaps for the child to respond.

Given the many obstacles children with autism face in processing information, it is likely that they will lose sight of the original issue. Practitioners need to develop a range of refocusing strategies which bring the child back to the initial challenge or task. These strategies may include scheduling the child to check the question at predetermined intervals, such as every three minutes. In other situations, practitioners may decide to regularly refocus the child on the task by verbal or gestural prompting. The difficulties faced by children with autism in processing information goes to the heart of the condition itself. Supporting children in this area requires sensitivity, knowledge of the condition and knowledge of the child.

Suggestion Box

1. Decide the key content of your lesson and write this down in bullet points.
2. Consider the least number of words you could use to deliver this key content.
3. Develop supportive materials for each phrase you plan to use.
4. Break up the content into stages of the lesson, allocating sufficient time for each phase to be delivered.
5. Decide how much time you will allow for a response before you will intervene.
6. Adjust as necessary to maintain momentum.

SUPPORTING COMMUNICATION

Impairment in the area of communication is one of the defining features of autism and often its most readily noticeable characteristic. The breadth of the autistic spectrum dictates that there is a range of difficulties in this area, including those children who are preverbal and communicate little or nothing through vocalisations, gesture or posture to others who appear to be linguistically fluent and in command of a large vocabulary. However, throughout the whole spectrum there are distinct and pervasive problems in the area of communication and whilst the degree of difficulty will vary, the existence of an impairment will be universal.

Our aim as practitioners must be threefold. Firstly, we must identify the communicative strategies the child uses, regardless of their current effectiveness. Secondly, we must focus on the ways in which we can support the child's existing communication strategies, valuing their efforts to communicate and ensuring that these efforts are productive and meaningful. Finally, we must develop the child's existing communication strategies further, enabling the child to increase the effectiveness of their communication.

A good starting point in this huge endeavour is to assume nothing. There is little in the behaviour of many people with autism which can conclusively and consistently inform us about their communication skills. There are people with autism who speak with apparent ease and elegance and yet cannot detect the subtleties and nuances of language; the unspoken words which account for so much of our communication. There are other people with autism who exhibit no expressive language and yet appear to comprehend the written word, whilst others may speak only intermittently at times of great anxiety or in response to rare phenomena. Therefore, we can take nothing for granted and must begin our work in this area with an acknowledgement that we are moving into a complex and intriguing field.

Recognition of this should prompt us to engage the services of specialists, namely speech and language therapists. A thorough assessment of a child's communication profile by a skilled and knowledgeable specialist is a prerequisite for effective practice with children with autism. Failure to obtain such an assessment may lead to the use of inappropriate strategies and force us into the cardinal sin of assumption. Unfortunately, locating a specialist with the time, training and tools in order to conduct meaningful assessment is rarely straightforward. As we discussed before, doing nothing is not an option, therefore, practitioners need to be developing approaches which serve the needs of the child and can, when circumstances allow, be dovetailed into an evidence based programme of intervention devised by a specialist. Speech and language therapy services can be contacted either through the local education authority or local NHS trusts.

Approaches must be based on a structured period of observation and consultation in order to determine how a child is attempting to communicate.

Information should be acquired across a number of settings; children with autism invariably operate in different ways in different contexts. A variety of methods for collecting information is advisable in order to capture the complexity of the child. Video recordings of the child are particularly powerful as they enable us to spot the minutiae of the child's behaviour and identify factors which we do not always perceive when we are with the child. Interviews with parents, siblings, transport assistants, former teachers, lunch-time assistants, indeed anyone who is a part of the child's life will help build up a picture of the child's communication profile. Finally, direct observations need to be spread over a defined period of time in order to track any changes and adaptations which are occurring in the child's communicative efforts. Observations should be structured and purposeful, designed for a specific reason and take place in a variety of settings. Where possible, a number of different people using a common format should conduct the observations in order to offer different perspectives and alternative understandings.

This period of observation and consultation should be defined at the outset and not drag on aimlessly. Moreover, if suitable strategies begin to emerge at any point, then implement them; don't wait until the end of the observation period if the child will benefit from them now. Once the period is complete, a repertoire of approaches should be implemented which are underpinned by principles and understandings recognised as fundamental to good communication practice for pupils with autism.

There must be a shared acknowledgement of the ephemeral nature of the spoken word. The spoken word lives for a fraction of a second, then disappears. If a person finds difficulty in processing spoken language, this creates major difficulties. For the child with autism, understanding words is like trying to catch a butterfly without a butterfly net. Some children may capture the odd word or syllable – giving half-meanings, and allowing partial interpretation. Others, will catch nothing that is said and grasp at the empty air for meaning.

Our challenge as practitioners is to give permanence to words. This can be achieved through three major channels. The first of these is familiarity, achieved by the consistent and limited use of a prescribed vocabulary in specified settings. Secondly, we can build structure around words, using music, rhyme or set phrases to give form to language. Finally, we can utilise the strengths many people with autism have in the visual field by employing visual materials to support spoken language. This can be in the form of pictures, symbols, photographs or writing depending on the individual and the context. Remember, irrespective of cognitive ability or apparent command of language, there will be some form of communication impairment and therefore, the need to develop strategies to support the child's understanding and use of language.

Considering the experience of failure in communication shared by many children with autism, it is not surprising that the language environment can be aversive and threatening. None of us like doing things we are not good at and most of us avoid failure by not addressing our shortcomings. For many people with autism, the spoken word is just a barking dog – relentless, meaningless and oppressive. Ironically, the education system is populated by talkative people, skilled communicators, who enjoy using language and exploring ideas through this medium. Consequently, there is the potential for a clash of cultures if practitioners are not able to adapt the use of language to the culture of the child.

Language use must be tailored to the needs of the child. It must be concrete, literal and direct. Take time to reflect on the amount of spoken language you use and then consider how much language you need to use. Is it possible to say what you need to say using fewer words? Think of the language environment as your classroom in which words are the resources and objects in your room. Just as good practice thrives in a classroom environment that is well laid out, where resources are clearly labelled and logically arranged, so too the language environment needs to be tidy, clutter-free and, above all, functional. We wouldn't leave pencils, paint pots and plasticine lying all over the room and neither should we do so with words.

CASE STUDY

From the Chalkface ...

Lunch-times have always been a challenge. It seems that during lunch-time we lump together everything our children aren't too good at and ask them to get on with it. Not surprisingly, we were having a difficult half term settling new children into the lunch-time routine and staff were becoming downhearted.

So we did something. For a whole week, we had a member of staff sitting apart from the pupils and analysing the use of language in the dining hall. At the end of the week, we took away the results and discussed them as a team. Clearly, we were using too many words and so we made a concerted effort to cut down the amount of language used in key areas.

1 Adult–adult interaction. This was discouraged unless absolutely necessary. Staff were encouraged to devise a range of nods and winks in order to communicate with one another or asked to speak softly in order to obtain necessary items.

2 Child–adult interaction. This was supported entirely by visual materials and when children engaged adults in conversation they were encouraged to speak softly and for limited periods.

The effect of this change in approach was dramatic and immediate. It did not solve all our lunch-time problems; not all of these were caused by language difficulties. However, it did enable us to control one factor in the lunch-time context. The atmosphere became noticeably calmer. Adults were able to identify potential difficulties more easily simply because they could hear themselves think. Children became more confident in their use of language because there was less language competition. It taught us more than any other single strategy we have recently employed; how crucial it is to get the language environment right.

Children with autism do not tend to instinctively orientate to the human voice. The sound of a human has no more relevance for them than other environmental sounds; passing cars, the banging of a door, the wind rustling through leaves. Therefore, unlike most of their peers, children with autism are not tuned in the moment the speaker begins to speak. Furthermore, people with autism do not automatically know that the language is being addressed to them. Whilst other children are able to utilise the body language of the speaker, the context of the interaction or the intonation used in order to determine whether language is addressed to them, the child with autism cannot draw upon of these instinctive cues. This results in the child apparently ignoring instructions or not responding to attempts at interactions from peers. It means that children with autism will often miss the important part of information being given because they aren't aware that the information is intended for them. All in all, it is a debilitating situation to be in and leaves the child at a huge disadvantage.

Once again, it is vital that the practitioner develops their practice to address the difficulties faced by the child. Many of the strategies are simple and straightforward; however, they do require us to get into good habits. The first example is simply to use the child's name at the beginning of any instruction or information being given. For example, rather than saying, 'Can everybody put things away now', it is better to identify the child specifically with the instruction, 'Jamila listen. Jamila put things away now please', before giving the instruction to the whole class. Remember, if you say, 'Put everything away now please Jamila', all Jamila is likely to hear is her name, followed by a rather confusing silence.

Another approach is to use visual cuing systems, such as coloured cards, to alert the child to the fact that something of significance to them is being said or symbols which ask the child to be quiet and listen. Similarly, music can be used to structure the beginning and end of sessions so that when the child hears a familiar refrain, they are aware that they need to listen for the next thing to do.

Recent advertisements publicising the work of the National Autistic Society have focused on the confusion caused by idiom in our use of language. Phrases such as 'eyes in the back of the head' or 'I'm all ears' are presented as examples of language use which, to the literally based child, is extremely bewildering, not to mention a little macabre! Unfortunately, practitioners are full of these sorts of maxims and sayings as they provide graphic commentary for many children and are a source of humour indicative of a strong adult–child relationship. However, they are likely to be unhelpful for many children with autism and potentially damaging to a significant few. Avoid using any such phrases and only employ humour if the child is likely to find it funny. Under no circumstances use sarcasm, irony or wit; it will be lost on the child and result in embarrassment all round.

Much of the meaning we convey in language is not carried by the words we use but rather by our posture, gesture, intonation and facial expression. These features can be as fleeting as words and are often misunderstood or just not noticed by people with autism. Furthermore, people with autism often exhibit idiosyncrasies in non-verbal communication which can, in themselves, be off-putting to others. Our aim as practitioners should be to limit the amount of confusion that our posture, gesture, intonation and facial expression can cause. This invariably requires us to become less effusive, less unpredictable (and, therefore, probably slower and calmer in our movements) and less reliant on the frowns and smiles that are effective currency with many of the children we teach. Try only using hand movements if you are indicating something and only use pointing if you are confident the child can follow the direction of the pointer. The stiller we can become as information givers, the less complex the information is for the child and the more likely that the information is interpreted correctly.

Finally, whatever stratagems are employed, whatever approaches engaged, it is of paramount importance that all parties working with the child are consistent and clear in their use. This can only be achieved if the strategies are arrived at through consensus and a shared understanding both of the reason for the adoption of the approach and the way in which the approach will operate. Consultation, trust and openness are prerequisites in the drive for consistency; consistency is an absolute requirement for the development of effective communication strategies for children with autism.

Supporting Communication: Dos

Do ...

✓ Recognise and value the child's communication strategies.

✓ Engage specialist support.

✓ Employ visual materials to support understanding.

✓ Use concrete, literal and precise language.

✓ Say the child's name before any directions or instructions.

✓ Be consistent.

✓ Allow time for processing.

Supporting Communication: Don'ts

Don't ...

✗ Make assumptions based on the child's use of language.

✗ Talk too much.

✗ Expect the child to know you are talking to him or her.

✗ Use metaphor or idiom without explaining it.

✗ Rely on body language and facial expression.

✗ Work in isolation.

DEVELOPING FLEXIBLE THINKING

In some respects, developing flexible thinking in a child with autism is the most challenging component of a practitioner's work. We can see what a child is doing with regard to communication or socialisation; we can quantify that according to a number of rating scales and plan our strategies accordingly. In the areas of communication and socialisation, we can develop approaches in line with established and credible models, and evaluate the effect of interventions by observing external outcomes. Flexible thinking, on the other hand, is by definition internalised and hidden.

Difficulties in the ability to think flexibly affects every aspect of the child's life. The development of communication and social understanding in a child with autism is invariably hampered by the child's inability to think flexibly, creating numerous obstacles to learning. Consequently, as practitioners, it is an area of the child's learning which we must address with urgency if we are to make real progress. Developing flexible thinking in a child with autism is perhaps the most challenging area of our work, but it is also potentially the most rewarding, enduring and empowering for the child.

Naturally, the breadth of the spectrum entails that the way in which an individual child's rigidity of thought shows itself will vary. There will be children who have an extremely circumscribed repertoire of behaviours: twiddling pieces of string, flapping their hands, humming set phrases from Disney cartoons. There will be children who display highly specialised knowledge of discrete areas: experts on dinosaurs, deep-sea trenches or Second World War militaria. There will be children who become hysterical if the car journey to school alters or become very angry if they are expected to do a job which is normally done by another child. Some children may shut down if there are unplanned changes in their lives, such as a supply teacher in class or the arrival of a new pet. Whatever the manifestation, the root cause is the same and the strategies we use as practitioners need to be developed with this impairment in mind.

Begin by trying get into the child's way of thinking. It is only by trying to understand the child's understanding that we can begin to formulate ideas about how we might develop more flexible patterns of thought. In practical terms this means starting where the child is. We know that one indicator of inflexible thinking can be seen in the child's lack of joint attention skills (Sigman et al., 1986). Many of us will have spent fruitless hours trying to draw the child into playing our games or sharing our interests. Experience shows that it is far more productive to begin by joining in the child's chosen activity and then developing that activity beyond its current confines. Aim for what is possible; this means gradually evolving an activity around the child's existing thought patterns. Be prepared to persevere, it may take many months before the child shows interest in things you are doing. Once again, video recording activities and interactions will enable you to detect some of the more fleeting moments of progress which you may otherwise miss.

Having involved yourself in what the child is doing, think of ways in which you can add another dimension to the activity. If the child twiddles string, can you introduce different types of string, different textures or colours? Can you encourage the child to use a different hand to play with the string or to share the string with you whilst you both play with it? If the child likes to talk about hover-crafts, can you extend the conversation to other types of transport or other types of boats? Could you learn about Christopher Cockerill or other inventions and inventors from the mid-twentieth century? Can you both extend and enhance the child's knowledge and thereby introduce more elasticity into the way in which the child thinks?

Another important element of practice in this area involves enabling the child with autism to better understand processes of change. It is widely acknowledged, almost to the extent of becoming a defining feature of the condition, that many people with autism do not cope well with change. This is potentially misleading. Like all of us, people with autism do not cope well with changes they cannot understand and it is this understanding which is impaired. Therefore, our efforts as practitioners should be directed towards helping the child to understand that a change is happening, why that change is happening, how it will happen and what will be the expected outcome.

In order to achieve this, it is good practice to build some element of change, something unpredictable, into the child's everyday routine. This enables the child to experience change within the secure context of their daily routine. It is advisable to ensure that these changes are small and, from your perspective, relatively insignificant – you may have to abandon the planned for change if the child reacts particularly adversely. Try altering things like the order in which you read the register, the tasks children are responsible for, the place people sit in the minibus or the circuit of activities laid out in the P.E. lesson. Prior to introducing the change:

- inform the child that there has been a change

- explain why this change has been made

- predict what will happen

- describe how things will turn out.

Naturally, the way in which these four points are covered will vary according to each child's needs and strengths.

Inform. This may take the form of verbal information, such as 'John, today there is a change. We will do Art before our numeracy session.' For other pupils it may be necessary to hold up a symbol showing 'Change' and draw the child's attention to this.

Explain. Change is generally difficult to explain as change is often the result of a chain of events which cannot be easily tracked. Indeed on occasion, you may not know yourself why the school hall is out of action. Your explanation may be verbal and should begin with a clear cueing word, such as 'because', so that your conversation with John may now be, 'John, today there is a change. We will do Art before our numeracy session. This is because Mrs Sullivan is coming in to help us with our numeracy and she cannot come until 10:30.' For other children you may have to use symbols or photographs, which will generally convey a less sophisticated message. However, such devices can be used to show that something is not available or someone is absent.

Predict. Predicting what will happen during the change will help the child to overcome their fear of the unknown and give a structure to events as they unfold. Here, both language and symbols are equally effective. Pictures and symbols can provide a scheduled sequence of events whilst a verbal commentary can guide the child through the expected change. Our conversation with John will now be, 'John, today there is a change. We will do Art before our numeracy session. This is because Mrs Sullivan is coming in to help us with our numeracy and she cannot come until 10:30. We will finish our artwork by 10:15, have outside play and then line up ready to go out of school. We are going to walk to up to the road in order to carry out a traffic census similar to the one we did in April.'

Describe. Describing intended outcomes enables the child to form a mental image of what is required and, therefore, to better understand when the change process is complete. Again images and language are equally powerful. Presenting a child with a picture of the final product or telling the child how things will be different once change is complete helps to resolve the whole process. John's information is now complete: 'John, today there is a change. We will do Art before our numeracy session. This is because Mrs Sullivan is coming in to help us with our numeracy and she cannot come until 10:30. We will finish our artwork by 10:15, have outside play and then line up ready to go out of school. We are going to walk to up to the road in order to carry out a traffic census similar to the one we did in April. When we are by the road Mrs Sullivan will help you count all the buses. You will come back to school at 11:15 and Mrs Sullivan will help you write all about the things you found out on the computer.'

Planning for change in this way not only enables the child to cope with the specific change that you are addressing but also to cope better with change as a concept. The child becomes accustomed to things not always adhering to set routines and learns that change does not necessarily equate to difficulties. The essential features of this approach are that it is based in a known context, populated by familiar people and is clearly explained in segmented parcels of information. As with other aspects of practice for children with autism, presenting this information visualy enhances their understanding.

A further aspect of developing flexible thinking involves encouraging pupils with autism to problem-solve. Opportunities may be incidental or intentional but practitioners must either seize the moment or contrive one in order to encourage the child to think adaptively and effectively. When presenting pupils with autism with problems to solve, an intricate balance between the support we give and freedom to fail must be found. This requires experience, professionalism and a comprehensive knowledge of the child. We must allow the child to make choices, sometimes the wrong choices, but not let them flounder in a frustrating fug. We need to encourage the child to try new things but not in such a way as to frighten them.

An effective way of achieving this is to work with the child to develop structures which enable them to problem-solve. You may discuss a series of scenarios with the child and provide them with a list of approaches to resolving those scenarios. Initially, these need to be very simple and guarantee success because it is essential that the child gains confidence in their ability to work in this way. An early example might be:

1   If you cannot find your pencil

2   Put your hand up

3   When Mr Saunders looks at you and says, 'Yes Hannah', you say

4   'Mr Saunders, I can't find my pencil'

5   Mr Saunders will bring a pencil to you.

This can be further developed to include incrementally more difficult challenges and less adult support. Consequently, the child will develop increasingly independent and adaptable behaviour which can be encouraged across a greater range of contexts.

For the child whose language skills would not support this approach, different challenges based on the same principles and focused on the same objectives can be introduced. For example, when setting out familiar tasks for the child, withhold particular items which the child needs. Provide the means for the child to obtain these items, such as symbols, pictures or written cue cards, but do not provide the item itself until a request is made. You may have to wait some time for the child to realise what is required; remember many children have learnt to depend on others to do everything for them. You may have to devise a cueing system to prompt the child; another adult might act as a model for requesting items.

Once this initial step has been achieved, the level of challenge can be gradually increased. Having requested the necessary item, children might not be presented with the item but told where to get the item from for themselves. Initially, this may be simply in a box on the table with the eventual objective that children locate items from storage cupboards in or near the classroom. It may be advisable, for the purposes of developing flexible thinking, to vary the place where items are stored so that the child cannot simply go to a cupboard and expect to find an item.

A final thought in this area relates to our practice and the way it may appear to the child with autism. We need to ask ourselves whether the child with autism thinks that we are inflexible thinkers. Are we rigid in the way we want things done, inflexible in our attachment to timetables or pedantic in our insistence on sameness? This is not offered to criticise the existence of regulation in our schools and classrooms but only to cause us to think about why we have such frameworks, what they do for us and how much we depend upon them. In reflecting on this we may come to a better understanding of why children with autism develop rigidities in their thinking and how, perhaps, it is not rigidity itself that is difficult for the learner with autism but rather the point at which their rigidity clashes with ours.

Chapter 6

Established and Effective Strategies

- Discusses the role of assessment in planning appropriate programmes for children with autism.

- Provides an overview of interventions used with pupils with autism including TEACCH, SPELL, PECS.

There is no magic to teaching children with autism. Successful practice for pupils with autism is the result of sound knowledge, hard work and appropriate resources. It is an extension and refinement of many basic pedagogic principles and is attainable to those practitioners who are able to adapt their practice and remain open to learning themselves. Whilst many people encountering pupils with autism for the first time will feel unskilled and in need of a complete over-haul of their practice, it is rarely the case that this is necessary. There will be the need to adjust to the culture of autism, to moderate certain elements of practice or enhance others, but the core qualities of a good practitioner are constant and apply to teaching children across all sectors and settings. So it is important that practitioners value themselves and their practice. It is crucial that we believe in ourselves if we want our children to believe in us. We don't expect to be right all the time or have a ready solution to every problem, but we must be secure in the knowledge that our practice and the approaches we employ are thoughtfully developed and open to improvement.

A central component of this is the need for practitioners to continuously evaluate their work and consider new ways and methods for extending their skills and knowledge. There is an abundance of interventions and approaches in the field of autism and identifying appropriate methods for individual pupils and contexts is seldom straightforward. The wealth of strategies available can be problematic; practitioners can be overwhelmed by the sheer number of differing, sometimes contradictory, approaches or seduced by one particular method to the exclusion of all others. As a result, the advantages of sound and effective interventions can be missed and opportunities for learning lost. Therefore, it is advisable for practitioners to develop a rationale for the approaches they select which combines an understanding of the child's learning needs and a knowledge of the theoretical and ethical basis of each approach.

As there is no magic to teaching pupils with autism, it is wise to treat any approach which lays claim to being a 'cure', or demands the exclusion of all other interventions, with scepticism. Good practitioners do not narrow their options or harbour unrealistic expectations. Autism is a lifelong condition which is manifest in as many different ways as there are individuals who experience it. Consequently, a cure is illusory and restricting practice to a single approach is unlikely to meet the range of needs encountered. Similarly, practitioners must guard against developing practice which is too eclectic and represents a patchwork of unsuitable and half-hearted measures.

The aim must be to develop practice which integrates approaches that have been identified as appropriate into a coherent, enduring and realistic programme for the child. To arrive at this point practitioners need to exercise their skills in and knowledge of:

- assessment

- interventions and approaches

- evaluation.

Each of these processes has an important role to play across all areas of life for the child with autism. However, for the purposes of this book, these terms are focused in the field of education and will not incorporate wider issues, such as diagnosis, medical intervention or life planning. For information regarding wider issues in the child's life refer to the **National Autism Plan for Children** (NIASA, 2003).

ASSESSMENT

Assessing the learning needs of children with autism can be difficult and frustratingly inconclusive. Ironically, it is these very features which tell us why assessment for children with autism is so important. Because many children with autism are complex, challenging and unsuited to standard assessments, practitioners need to engage in a comprehensive programme which represents the child's learning profile, determines their level of attainment and informs the planning of appropriate future objectives.

Purpose

A key feature of meaningful assessment is clarity of purpose. Practitioners must have clear and well founded objectives driving the assessment forward and defining the boundaries of the assessment process. These objectives may be seen as responses to a series of questions focusing on, for example:

- *What* do I want to find out?

- *Why* do I want to know this?

- *How* will I obtain this information?

- *Who* will be involved?

- *When* will the process start?

- *What* will I do with the information I obtain?

Combining the answers into a coherent response enables the practitioner to develop a rationale for assessment and a clear concept of how this will directly and positively affect the child's learning.

Perspectives

Given the complexity of children with autism, meaningful assessment must be based on the principles of triangulation. This is a term used by map-makers, and relates to the use of measurements taken from several different reference points in order to arrive at an accurate representation of the landscape (the term is also used in social research and refers to the practice of comparing and contrasting several sets of data to check for reliability and validity). If we wish to understand the 'learning landscape' of the child with autism, we must adopt a similar strategy. Practitioners involved in the assessment of children with autism need to employ a number of perspectives in order to build up a composite assessment of the child which recognises the complexity of the learner with autism. Practitioners need to take the following into account:

The Context. The child with autism is likely to perform in differing ways in different contexts. A meaningful assessment of the child must incorporate perspectives from the range of contexts the child experiences in order to achieve reliability and validity. It is important to bear in mind that people make up the context as much as the physical environment and, therefore, there is a need to incorporate information from a number of people in the assessment.

Variable Performance. The impact of autism on the child determines that performance during the process of assessment is likely to be compromised. The newness of the materials being encountered, the unfamiliarity of assessment conditions, the difficulties the child experiences in understanding what is required, are all common factors in skewing the results of assessment. However, this skew is in itself important data as it shows the difficulties the child is experiencing. For example, if a child cannot perform a task in one context, which he is known to be able to perform in another, this tells us something important about the barriers to learning the child encounters.

Irregular Learning Profile. Many, if not most, children with autism have irregular learning profiles. This means that their learning neither follows orthodox developmental pathways nor provides insights to a global view of the child's attainment. Intriguingly, many children with autism seem to achieve things that the conventional view of learning development would claim are impossible to attain without first having acquired skills the child does not appear to possess. Alternatively, these children do not have some basic skills which their level of attainment would suggest they should have. Assumptions of the child's overall ability based on evidence of their performance in specific areas are unhelpful. A child may be very able in some areas; other areas of the child's learning may be severely impaired. This disparity presents one of the greatest challenges to practitioners and determines that assessment must be based on several perspectives in order to see both the strengths and needs of the child.

Well-being. No child can be expected to perform well if they are tired, tense, ill or upset. Children with autism can be particularly prone to ill health either through associated conditions, such as epilepsy, the effect of a very restricted diet, poor sleep patterns or the consequence of living under stress for much of the time. Assessment which takes place across a range of settings and over a period of time may allow some of these issues to be evened out. It may also show that these states are enduring and influential features on the child's learning.

Methods

Having established both the purpose and perspectives of assessment, practitioners need to consider which assessment methods are going to be of most value. Methods can be characterised in several ways. There are those methods which are based on formalised, standardised approaches and those which take place under everyday, less formal situations. There are methods which are lead by specialists, such as educational psychologists or speech and language therapists, using specific assessment instruments. There are methods which involve parents and practitioners in an evolving dialogue of practice. Each of these has a distinct purpose and a particular value. Each of these will tell us something different about the child and deepen our understanding of his/her learning. Across this range, methods may involve:

- observation

- interviews

- test materials

- checklists,

some of which are designed specifically for children with autism, whilst others are more generic to child development.

Such diversity is necessary and appropriate given the range of needs encountered on the autistic spectrum and the variety of contexts within which children, their families and practitioners operate. Our task as practitioners is to determine which combination of methods suits the purpose we have defined and offers a number of valid perspectives of the child. There are several well-established assessment tools which may help practitioners in developing their understanding of the child. Amongst the more common ones used in the field are the:

- Psychoeducational Profile – Revised (Schopler et al., 1990)

- Early Years Observation Profile (Cumine et al., 2000)

- Assessment and Intervention Schedule (Aarons and Gittens, 1992)

- Pre-Verbal Communication Schedule (Kiernan and Reid, 1987)

- The Pragmatic Profile of Early Communication Skills (Dewart and Summers, 1988)

However, practitioners must not underestimate the contribution of their own practice-based observations and professional insight to the assessment process. By combining formal methods, close collaboration with the child's family and the practitioner's gradually acquired knowledge of the child, the assessment process can provide a firm foundation for the planning of an effective and relevant learning programme for the child.

The final stage in the assessment process involves determining how our understanding of the child's learning will be incorporated into the child's learning programme. It is essential at this point that the information obtained through the assessment period is shared with all relevant parties. Effective planning for children with autism is collaborative. Consequently, there must be a shared understanding of the child amongst everyone involved in producing the child's learning programme. This is best achieved by bringing people together at a **Learning Planning Meeting** in which the assessment period is discussed and the child's future programme is considered.

> ### Suggestion Box
>
> At the outset of the assessment period, set a date for the Learning Planning Meeting. Invite people who have a direct input into the child's life including the child themselves where appropriate, parents and other close family members, practitioners working with the child, specialists, such as speech therapists and education psychologists, social workers, care workers and health professionals. Invite people to prepare a contribution to the meeting based on their observations and assessments. For some professionals, the Data Protection Act restricts the information they are able to share; you may wish to circumvent this by consulting with parents or the young person prior to the meeting date.
>
> Prepare some initial ideas for the child's learning programme based on your assessments. Adjust and adapt these during the meeting in the light of the information shared. Aim to have finalised the child's programme within a week of the meeting. Ensure that assessment becomes cyclical, building into your programme evaluative processes and review dates.

INTERVENTIONS AND APPROACHES

Effective intervention programmes for children with autism are based upon a sound theoretical understanding of the condition supported by reputable and robust research. For the practitioner new to the field of ASDs, the number and range of interventions available can seem overwhelming and the apparent contradictions between approaches can be confusing. Perhaps the best advice on offer is to stick to the tried and tested, both in terms of the strategies considered and the sources of information investigated. Whilst this may seem conservative, it will save the practitioner reinventing any wheels or buying into unproven and spurious interventions. In discussing the range of treatments available, the NAPC cautions:

> Therapies as diverse as swimming with dolphins, being swung around in nets, dosing with evening primrose oil or listening to tapes of filtered sound have all been suggested as effective. However, recent reviews have generally indicated that many of these claims are made in the absence of any scientific data.
>
> (NIASA, 2003)

This advice must prompt us all to carefully consider which approaches we adopt or endorse.

There are strategies and approaches which have worked well for many children with autism over a number of years. Within this group there is usually a way forward for the child, often by integrating interventions focused on the child's specific needs. Although there is no one intervention or approach that is right for all children with autism, there are features common to this core group which are known to be important to people with autism. These include:

- structure – in practice, procedures and the physical environment

- clarity – in purpose, expectations and outcomes

- consistency – across environments and between people

- modification – of practice and the environment to the culture of autism

- acceptance – of the culture of autism, its differences and strengths.

Although there is diversity amongst established and effective interventions, they work because they recognise the need for these components to be evident in the programme. Sometimes these features are not immediately apparent, but they will be found, to some extent, within each intervention which has a proven record for people with autism.

Structured Teaching within TEACCH

The approach most widely associated with autism is known as **TEACCH** (**T**reatment and **E**ducation of **A**utistic and related **C**ommunication handi-capped **CH**ildren), which developed from the work of Eric Schopler and colleagues during the 1960s. TEACCH is a whole life approach for people with autism that promotes the principles which underpin the structured teaching approach developed within the programme. These principles are based on a recognition of the characteristic strengths and impairments of people with autism. Strengths are typically:

- special interests

- rote memory skills

- visual processing

- attention to detail

- affinity for routine.

Whereas, impairments are generally found in the areas of:

- verbal expression

- auditory processing

- high distractability

- organisational skills

- generalisation of skills

- difficulty with change.

Understanding of these features evolved into the structured teaching approach used within TEACCH.

The four major components of structured teaching in the TEACCH program are:

- physical organisation
- schedules
- work systems
- task organisation.

(Schopler and Mesibov, 1995)

In broad terms these components can be seen to represent the where, when, what and how of the child's learning; supporting understanding through structure, consistency and focus on the child's characteristic strengths.

The physical organisation relates to the layout of the classroom and other relevant learning areas, including the school hall, shared play and activity areas, toilets and bathrooms, dining areas and playgrounds. The objective is to provide clearly demarcated areas for specific activities so that the child learns to associate x place with x activity. These areas are signalled to the child by employing words, symbols and photographs to describe the purpose of the area. A further feature of these areas can be the use of colour to indicate a change in purpose or function for an area. For example, a table top used for group work, becomes the snack table when it is covered with a green tablecloth.

A central feature of the physical organisation of the classroom, is the use of a transition area. The transition area responds to the difficulty people with autism have in understanding change and, therefore, provides an information point at which all details of change are displayed. The transition area is where schedules are located and where children are shown the next activity in which they will be involved.

Another aspect of the physical environment relates to the sensory stimulus within the classroom. Children with autism generally benefit from a physical environment which is structured so as to reduce the potential for distraction or over-stimulation. This does not mean that rooms should be bare and soulless, but rather that attention should be given to developing environments which are 'optimally stimulating' (Jordan and Powell, 1995). Naturally, this will vary from child to child and context to context; indeed in many situations, practitioners will need to balance the needs of each child in the class group in order to arrive at this point. However, for the child with autism to learn effectively, the practitioner must consider ways in which sensory stimuli can be diminished in order to enable the child to focus on the relevant aspects of the learning activity.

In many classrooms which accommodate children with autism, dividers are used to reduce visual or auditory distractions. These may be cupboards, work units or standard office dividers and are used to define a work-station for the

Figure 6.1 **Transition Area**

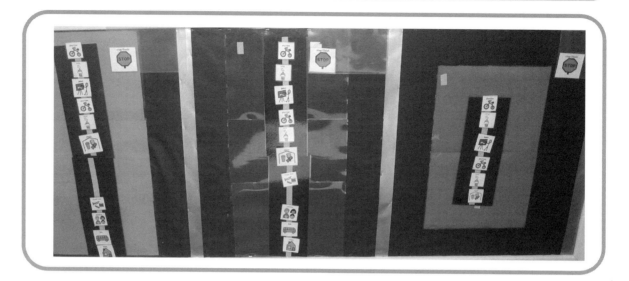

child within which all potentially distracting elements are diminished. In autism specific environments several such work-stations may be found in a classroom; in the non-specialist setting, a single work-station may be developed within the general classroom.

For many children with autism, noise can be both highly distracting and frightening. Adopting a low-level noise approach is generally advisable, promoting a calm and quiet atmosphere within the classroom. In the mainstream environment this is not always easily attainable. Where this is the case, it can be useful to encourage the child with autism to wear headphones either to muffle environmental sound or to allow them to listen to relaxing music. Practitioners also need to consider the potential for distraction caused by noises that people without autism will automatically filter out. For example, if the classroom is too near the staff car park, children may lose their focus every time an engine starts. Other children with autism will be distracted by the flow of water through the heating pipes, the barely perceptible tick of the classroom clock or the music lesson from the classroom next to yours. Some of these factors can not be eradicated, yet with careful and creative thinking the effect of these distractions can be reduced.

We also need to be aware of sensory stimuli other than visual or auditory distractions which may impede pupils with autism. Many use their sense of smell to investigate items. Smells which can be pleasant to others may be strongly off-putting to a person with a heightened sensitivity in this area. Perfumes, aftershaves, soaps and shampoos can all be either over-stimulating or positively aversive to certain children. The classroom itself will consist of many smells which we may have got used to, but the child with autism will not be able to ignore. Thought may need to be given to glues, paints, plants and even cleaning materials used in the classroom.

Directly related to this sensory channel, is the sense of taste. Children with autism may exhibit behaviour, such as mouthing or licking objects, which may be inappropriate or dangerous. Some children experience a condition known as **pica** which involves the ingestion of non-edible materials and can be extremely detrimental to the child's health. However, some children are repulsed by tastes which others may find enjoyable and will, therefore, find places and activities associated with that taste, such as the dining hall or snack table, extremely aversive.

In addition to this, many children with autism find tactile sensations very stimulating or are highly tactile defensive. Some children love to rub their hands on the surfaces of desks or chairs or sense the coolness of windows against their cheek. Others find the feel of paper horrible or the squelch of finger paint repugnant. Whatever the circumstances, whatever the sensory channel, practitioners need to eliminate those components of the environment which distract the child from purposeful and productive learning.

Another aspect of the physical organisation of the learning environment relates to the relative location of rooms and the location of items within the room. Naturally, it is commonsense to locate rooms close to other environments relevant to the child's learning. For example, if a child is learning to use the toilet, it is sensible to make sure that his classroom is near to the toilet area. Or, if a child is involved in a frequent physical exercise programme, it may be helpful to place him in a classroom near to the school hall or with easy outside access. Similarly, the materials the child requires for learning must be accessible and located in a place that will not itself be distracting to the child. Over time, the distance between the child and the materials can be gradually increased in order to encourage independence, or changed in order to facilitate flexible thinking.

In developing the physical layout of the learning environment, practitioners need to think creatively and critically. For the child with autism, consideration of the physical layout of the room incorporates the obvious and the subtle, the concrete and the ambient. We need to audit the effectiveness of the learning environment's physical layout from the perspective of the child and not assume it to be effective because it resembles our concept of effective.

The second essential component of the TEACCH approach is the use of schedules: a sequenced visual timetable of the events and activities of the child's day. The precise presentation of the schedule will vary in detail depending on the child's cognitive ability and experience of using them. For children with a limited cognitive ability, objects of reference may be used to denote the forthcoming activity, such as a toothbrush being presented to enable the child to predict it is time to clean teeth. More commonly, children may use a strip of symbols or photographs to sequence events. More able individuals will carry diaries providing written information of the expectations of the day, week or month. Whatever the presentation, the enduring principles will remain the same.

Figure 6.2 Schedules

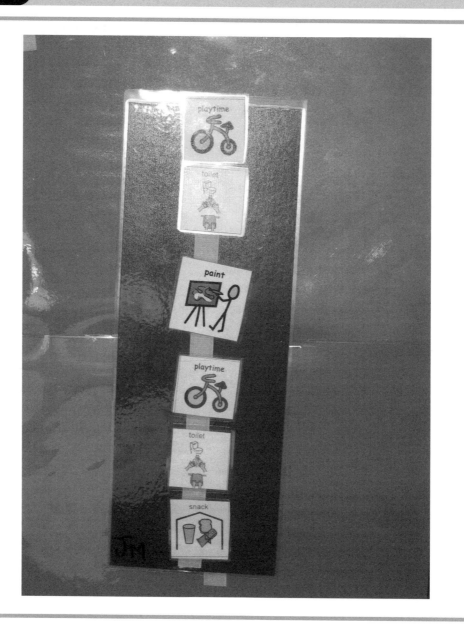

The use of schedules is a response to the difficulties children with autism have in understanding when activities and events will take place. Schedules compensate for the problems they face in spanning and sequencing time and are designed to enable the child to predict events and structure their day. Essentially, schedules organise time for children with autism without depending upon language skills, which may be lacking or inconsistent. They are visual reminders which encourage independence by structuring time in a clear, sequential manner. As each task or activity is completed, it is removed from the schedule, showing it has passed and indicating the next task in the order. The use of the schedule can be self-motivating in that it is predictable and reliable, and seems to give many children a sense of satisfaction and security.

Schedules can vary in their time span from a few seconds to extended periods. They can be used to outline the events of the school day or the sequential steps for a specified task. Presentation may be horizontal or vertical and may relate to whole class activities, individual pupils or both. Schedules might be fixed to a certain point or be transferable; carried around by the child in a diary-like format. Schedules can be devised by the practitioner in conjunction with the child, allowing the development of skills in negotiation and ensuring the child understands that the schedule brings with it rewards as well as demands.

The use of schedules is a transferable skill. Once the child has become used to the concept and has learnt to trust its structure and reliability, the schedule can be used to enable learning in a range of contexts. For example, a schedule depicting a dressing sequence can be used in the familiar context of the changing area in the school. Once the skill is established here, the schedule can be used to transfer the skill to the changing rooms in the public swimming baths or to support the child's dressing skills at home. Similarly, children who are anxious about the predictability of events outside the regular routine of school time, such as weekends or school holidays, can have schedules developed for use at home, describing the activities and events of the day.

The third key component of the TEACCH approach is the use of work systems. Well designed work systems give clear information to children about what is expected of them during a task and are essential in enabling children to develop greater independence during lesson time. They teach a child to work systematically and with purpose and share the advantage of being visually based thereby avoiding any obstacles associated with the child's communication difficulties.

Within a standard TEACCH model, tasks are presented to pupils in boxes or trays so that the child can easily see the items they will be working with. A strip with information corresponding to the study boxes is placed strategically on the child's desk. The study boxes are arranged to the left of the child in the order the child will be expected to complete them, which matches the corresponding information strip. This informs the child of the amount of work there is to be completed and the order in which it should be done. Crucially, the work system incorporates a finish box, where all completed tasks are placed. This is located to the right of the child and enables the child to see when they have completed their work. The sense of completion is important for many people with autism and work systems, like schedules, can become self-motivating, providing the child with a rewarding sense of satisfaction. Work systems can be adapted to suit the cognitive capacity of the child. Sometimes objects might be used to match the task in the study box. Other children may find a corresponding symbol system helpful, using coloured shapes or pictures they find motivating, such as animals, transportation or favourite cartoon characters. Some children will be able to understand and use a numerical or alphabetical system whilst others will be able to read whole words describing the task they are scheduled to complete.

The final component of the TEACCH system is task organisation. This refers to what might be seen as instructions for completing tasks, or 'jigs', to use the terminology employed by the programme. Like other components of TEACCH, jigs can be adapted to meet the developmental needs of the individual and may range from objects which model the required end result to written instructions on how to reach the final objective of the task. Jigs are intended to encourage the child with autism to look for instructions to guide their efforts. Developing this skill has important implications for the acquisition of new skills in later life and enables the child to generalise their skills to a range of settings.

An enduring feature of structured teaching is its capacity to enable people with autism to engage in learning opportunities which would otherwise be difficult for them to access. The challenge of accessing the National Curriculum for the UK has been addressed by Gary Mesibov and Marie Howley (Mesibov and Howley, 2003) as they discuss ways in which an evolving National Curriculum and a powerful inclusion agenda can provide opportunities for the implementation of approaches focused on the needs of children with autism:

> If pupils with ASD are to be successfully included it is essential that their learning needs and styles are recognised. The National Curriculum now paves the way for teachers to adopt a more flexible approach to the curriculum in relation to both appropriateness of content and methods of delivery.
>
> (Mesibov and Howley, 2003: 18)

This ability to respond to changes in the general context has enabled the structured teaching methods within TEACCH to remain effective and adaptable tools for practitioners. The focus on the core strengths and needs of the learner with autism, coupled with a practicality based on real life experiences, places TEACCH at the heart of many successful practitioner's practice.

SPELL

In the UK, best practice in the schools run by the National Autistic Society (**NAS**) was brought together under a common framework known by the acronym SPELL. This stands for:

- Structure

- Positive approaches and expectations

- Empathy

- Low arousal

- Links.

From these principles successful strategies can be developed. The NAS describe the SPELL approach as 'the common thread running through all of the specialist services provided by the National Autistic Society' (www.nas.org.uk). which underpins practice in all areas. Further information on this approach can be obtained through the NAS.

PECS

During the last decade, the introduction of the **P**icture **E**xchange **C**ommunication **S**ystem has made an incalculable contribution to the lives of many people with autism. PECS (Bondy and Frost, 2002; Frost and Bondy, 1994) is a communication system developed by Lori Frost and Andy Bondy in the 1980s based on their work with young children with autism (Frost and Bondy; 2002). As with TEACCH, PECS focuses on the characteristic features of the learner with autism capitalising upon visual strengths and a capacity for learning systematically whilst accommodating the difficulties caused by impairments in receiving, processing and expressing language.

PECS is incremental in its design, taking the learner through six phases, namely:

1   Phase One – initiating communication

2   Phase Two – expanding the use of pictures

3   Phase Three – choosing the message in PECS

4   Phase Four – introducing the sentence structure in PECS

5   Phase Five – teaching answering simple questions

6   Phase Six – teaching commenting.

(Bondy and Frost, 2002).

An essential feature of PECS is the permanence of the information being exchanged. The spoken word disappears as soon as it is spoken; gesture and facial expression are similarly short-lived. For the child with autism, who takes time to process information or has difficulty accessing words or phrases, PECS provides a constant visual source of information. This supports the child's understanding and, therefore, promotes successful communication opportunities. As communication becomes an increasingly positive experience for the child, so the child becomes more likely to engage in positive communicative interactions, creating a virtuous spiral of successful communication.

Verbal prompts are not used in PECS. This prevents the child from becoming prompt dependent and encourages spontaneity in communicative efforts. PECS places the initiative for communication with the child, promoting and sustaining the motivation necessary for communication to succeed. It enables the child to generalise skills to a range of contexts because many of the items used in PECS are portable so that the child is able to take supportive materials from place to place and person to person. This in turn allows communication to take place in a variety of contexts. For example, a child might learn to ask for a drink in the familiar setting of the classroom, then transfer this skill to the school dining hall and, eventually, be able to request a drink in a local café or restaurant.

For many children with autism, PECS provides a successful strategy for communication. Communicative acts become effective and motivating; a positive means to a positive end for the child. For those children who do not acquire any spoken language, PECS offers an alternative to never being able to express wants and needs. For children whose language is limited, PECS can act as a scaffold which supports language development and encourages increasing language skills. For some children, PECS becomes redundant as they develop sufficient skills to no longer require its augmentation. Whatever the specific detail, the impact of PECS on the learning and lifestyle of many children with autism has been both positive and enduring.

Minimal Speech Approach

A minimal speech approach (Potter and Whittaker, 2001) recognises the potentially aversive affect of complex language on children with autism. Therefore, the approach offers strategies for modifying the type and degree of speech used with children, focusing on key words and avoiding complex language structures. Many children with autism rely heavily on situational clues and daily routines to enhance their understanding of language. This can create a false impression of their ability to process language, leading to an inappropriate use of language by the adults around them. Phrases, such as 'Come on Terry put your coat on, the blue one, 'cause it's raining and that's got a hood on it. Oh, and remember, zip it up properly,' may result in Terry putting on, and successfully zipping up, his blue raincoat. But if we analyse what Terry has actually processed from this phrase it may only be the words 'coat on'. Terry may have noticed that it is raining, know from past experience that he wears his blue coat when it rains and understand he must zip it up to keep dry. However, when Terry appears in his zipped up blue coat, the adult may presume that Terry associates the word blue with the colour blue and knows what a hood is or understands what raining means. When these skills do not appear in other contexts, the adult may believe that Terry is being obstructive or resistant. As a consequence of this misjudgement, far too much language is used with the child and the key words the child might have been able to process are lost in the noise of words. This can lead to the child becoming anxious and opting out of using language, missing out altogether on opportunities for verbal communication.

Carol Potter and Chris Whittaker recommend the creation of a 'communication-enabling environment' (Potter, and Whittaker, 2001: 32) through the use of the following key features:

- reducing the use of speech in all situations

- appropriate mapping of single words

- giving information in non-verbal ways

- minimising 'running commentaries'

- delaying the use of speech when teaching new tasks

- avoiding temporal terms (today, tomorrow, yesterday) as early comprehension goals.

As practitioners, our natural reaction to a child who does not understand what we are saying is to try and explain more, use more language, give more detail. However, for children with autism, less is definitely more. The reduction of language enables the child to grasp the key components of the information and focus on what is understood.

Intensive Interaction

Intensive interaction is an approach pioneered by Melanie Nind and Dave Hewett which helps people with severe learning difficulties to develop skills in interaction and communication (Nind and Hewett, 1994; Nind and Hewett, 2001). The focus on these two key areas means that the intervention has many applications for people with autism, particularly those who also experience learning difficulties.

This approach is based on the principles of parent–baby interaction. During the first months of life, babies are frequently involved in pleasurable and rewarding interactions with adult care providers. Adults instinctively respond to the actions of the baby, giving meaning to the baby's actions and building these actions into a familiar repertoire of activities and games. As the child develops and the interactions increase and expand, relationships are strengthened and the basis of the child's future learning is formed. If this natural, instinctive process is disrupted through the child experiencing learning difficulties or impairments, opportunities for the development of skills are restricted. Consequently, the child may not acquire the prerequisite skills for social interaction and communication. Moreover, the actions of the baby have a profound influence on the adult's response. Therefore, if the child's development is problematic, it is likely to shape the action of an adult in a way which does not promote effective interactions.

Intensive interaction aims to encourage successful interactions by providing opportunities for individuals to engage in the type of reciprocal activity typical of infants and their caregivers. This includes developing an individual's understanding of the fundamentals of communication, such as turn-taking, eye contact and sharing attention. This is achieved by the practitioner applying the principles of parent–baby interaction through:

- being available for interaction

- establishing a relaxed and happy ambience

- allowing the individual to take the lead

- creating space and time for responses

- giving meaning to the individual's actions and responding appropriately

- developing a familiar pattern and routine to the repertoire of actions

- extending actions and interactions.

For some people with autism, the progress made through intensive interaction has both improved the individual's quality of life and contributed to the acquisition of new skills in the areas of interaction and communication. Practitioners who develop their skills and knowledge in intensive interaction are able to apply aspects of the approach to other areas of their practice. For example, practitioners become more tuned in to the child, noticing the subtle, often fleeting, cues and clues the child gives as precursors to interactive activity or readiness to respond. Importantly, practitioners who are skilled in intensive interaction are often sensitive to the amount of time a child needs to process information and judge the pauses between interactions with great skill.

Musical Interaction

Another powerful intervention which has many parallels with intensive interaction is musical interaction (Prevezer, 1990; Wimpory, 1995). Through this approach, the difficulties children with autism face in social timing are addressed using music to encourage the development of preverbal joint attention skills.

Initially, the child's spontaneous actions and sounds are treated as intentionally communicative. The adult responds using music as a way of joining in with the child, commenting on the child's actions or shaping the activity. For example, if a child is tapping the surface of a table, the adult may join in with the activity, introduce a song to the rhythm of the tapping and sing a lyric to a familiar tune which comments on the activity, such as:

Tanya taps the table top, table top, table top,
Tanya taps the table top, my fair lady,

to the tune of 'London Bridge'.

The natural structures of music provide a framework for the development of critical interaction skills in the child, including:

- sharing attention

- awareness of the communicative affect of their actions

- responding to pauses

- anticipating routines.

The familiarity of favourite songs, the enjoyment of the music itself and the non-invasive nature of the approach encourage the child to engage in interactions which they otherwise find difficult. Practitioners do not need to be music specialists to use this approach; singing or clapping rhythms are just as motivating to many children as is the skilled playing of an instrument. The approach draws the child into interaction through a shared enjoyment of music, developing not only important communication skills but also aspects of the child's self-esteem and self-image.

Play–Drama Intervention

Play–Drama intervention (Sherratt and Peter, 2002) offers a structured approach to developing play and imagination in children with autism. The approach takes as its starting point the generally held view that children learn through their play. Play enables the child to explore, experiment and discover; it provides them with opportunities to practice and refine skills and promotes creativity, empathy and social cohesion. However, given the fundamental impairments of autism, for many children with the condition this playfulness remains latent. These problems are potentially worsened by the tendency to concentrate solely on approaches which focus on the child's relative strength in logical, sequential tasks. This narrows opportunities to exercise the child's creative and playful potential despite the fact that:

> Logic would seem to suggest that children experiencing difficulty in a particular area (in this case, play) should receive more support in it, not less!
>
> (Sherratt and Peter, 2002: 3)

Dave Sherratt and Melanie Peter argue that engaging a developmental approach to play–drama intervention provides structures that enable the child to bring together logical and emotional processes, which it is felt people with autism have difficulty in integrating. By bringing together the rational and creative components of their understanding, the child acquires a more 'coherent understanding' (Sherratt and Peter, 2002: 20). The structures can be gradually broadened to incorporate increasingly complex play behaviour which ultimately contributes to the child's understanding of the wider world around them.

The approach identifies three key conditions for providing purposeful play experiences for children with autism, namely:

1 structure

2 interests

3 affect

and offers the view that children with autism need to be enabled and motivated in order to engage in play. Fundamental to the whole process is the interaction with sensitive adults.

As with other interventions, the early child–adult model of interactions, which are predictable and based on joint attention and shared meaning, provides a basis for initial activities. These are built on incrementally by rewarding desired play-acts until the child is involved in play which is both complex and sophisticated. The noticeable benefits of this approach include:

- progress in language skills

- improved social understanding

- advances in play skills to include symbolic, pretend and socio-dramatic play

- increased ability to cope with change

- reduced obsessive and repetitive behaviours

- developments in empathetic understanding

- increased spontaneity and creativity.

Whilst the cornerstones of this approach may seem contrary to the needs of a child experiencing the characteristic difficulties of autism, an argument can be made for directly addressing those difficulties through a structured programme based on sound theory and robust evidence. The potential benefits of the approach must prompt practitioners to consider how to incorporate play–drama intervention into the child's overall learning programme.

Social Stories

Social stories (Gray, 1994a, b; Gray and White, 2002) are designed to provide a person with autism with the social information they require to cope in a given situation. Developed in 1991 by Carol Gray, social stories either describe situations which are proving difficult for a person with autism or acknowledge the success and achievement of a person with autism using a format which is both sensitive to the perspective of the person and meaningful to them.

Gray describes social stories as a 'process' and a 'product'. The process involves the author of the story considering the situation from the perspective of the person with autism and writing a product using text and illustration in a way that is meaningful to the person. The story itself is specifically defined according to prescribed guidelines, namely:

1 descriptive – statements of fact

2 perspective – describing other people's internal states

3 affirmative – expressing generally shared values

4 directive – identifying suggested or recommended responses.

The ratio with which these sentence types are used is also clearly prescribed with between two and five descriptive/perspective/affirmative sentences being used for each directive sentence.

The positive and sensitive nature of social stories coupled with their clear structure and individual focus enable many children with autism to overcome a range of complex and confusing situations. The permanence of the text and illustrations allows the child to revisit the story in order to consolidate developing concepts, whilst the simple sentence structure enables the child to memorise key phrases, or mini-mantras, to recite when encountering potential difficulties.

EVALUATION

Just as assessment for a child with autism is often difficult, so too is evaluating the effectiveness of interventions and approaches. This is often because of the number of variables involved in the child's life at any one time and the possible effects, good and bad, that these variables may have.

Nevertheless, we need to continuously evaluate the effectiveness of our practice and define milestones at which we regularly review the child's progress. There are likely to be formal, statutory points at which this review is required, however, good practice determines the frequency with which we review a child's progress, is responsive to the child's needs and the context in which we are working.

The approaches described above lend themselves to continuous evaluation. They are generally incremental in design and phased in their application. Consequently, practitioners naturally arrive at points at which they consider the progress the child has made and whether they are ready for the next stage. This is a strength of these established strategies and can be used to guide practitioners through difficult components of their practice.

As a general rule, evaluation should involve the practitioner in a series of questions asking:

- What progress has the child made?

- What progress had I expected the child to make?

- What factors are currently affecting the child?

- What affect have the approaches used with the child had?

- How effectively are we using these approaches?

- How skilled are we in these approaches?

- What other strategies might benefit the child?

In evaluating the progress of the child, we are invariably evaluating our own effectiveness as practitioners. For this process to be beneficial, we must be honest, fair and open to necessary change.

Chapter 7

Sharing Good Practice

Presents ten lesson templates to be used as part of a reflective process by practitioners.

The following lesson templates have been contributed by experienced practitioners from the field of ASDs who were asked to share lessons which they felt had been particularly successful, and identify the crucial elements of the lesson which had contributed to its effectiveness. The purpose of this exercise is to provide practitioners with concrete examples of the ways in which our knowledge of how children with autism learn has been applied to the real world of the classroom. The templates are not intended as 'off-the-peg' lessons, but rather as reference points to support practitioners in developing practice. Essentially, the templates should encourage people to reflect on the approaches they use and determine whether the key issues for children with autism are securely embedded in their practice. The use of the templates is fluid. A person might use the template on English to reflect upon their practice in the area of, let us say, ICT, or take the session on Music as a starting point for developing their practice in Science. Each child is unique, each learning situation specific to itself, therefore, we cannot transplant practice. However, we can share principles and ask ourselves, 'What is it about this lesson that made it a success?' or 'How can I apply that to my current situation?'

These resources are also available to download from the PCP website (www.paulchapmanpublishing.co.uk/resources/hanbury.pdf).

Communication

Learning Objectives	• to acknowledge the presence of others, • to cooperate with simple requests, and • to attend to the activity for a short period of time.
About the Group	Six pupils aged between five and seven. All children with statements of SEN (Special Educational Needs) specifying ASDs compounded by SLD (Severe Learning Difficulties). One child using one word level, all other children preverbal. High staff to pupil ratio (3:6). All children display some degree of challenging behaviour. Varied personalities in the group balance each other well. Children are beginning to anticipate the routine of the lesson.
Context	Lesson delivered as part of regular daily circle time.
Approaches	TEACCH; PECS; Planned Behaviour Support.
Resources	Laminated visual aids; white magnetic board; tape recorder.
Environment	Children seated in semi-circle, facing display board. Cupboards and screens are used to block out distractions and define group area.
Content	• A 'Hello Song' is sung to each child in turn. Each child stands in front of the group with adult support whilst 'Hello …' is sung to them. • Child responds by waving/acknowledging group appropriately. • Child finds picture of themselves from selection of others displayed on a photo board. • Picture is removed from board and placed onto main display board under the correct day of the week.
Contingency	All children are required to stay with the group throughout the session. If a child becomes significantly challenging they may be removed to another adult directed activity.
Discussion	The learning objectives of this lesson show **high expectations** for this dependent and challenging group of young children. The objectives are achieved by using highly visual resources presented in a **low distraction** environment. The regular, predictable **routine** of the session and familiarity of the resources used further supports the children's learning. Crucially, there is a **contingency** plan which ensures that any challenging behaviour is comparatively ineffective. If the situation becomes such that a child needs to leave the group, an alternative adult directed activity is ready for use. Differentiation is achieved through the different responses required of each child and through **subtle variations** in the presentation of photographs.

Educating Pupils with Autistic Spectrum Disorders © Martin Hanbury, 2005

English

Learning Objectives	- to take an active part in a story-telling session, - to develop self-advocacy skills, and - to attend an activity in a group setting.
About the Group	Three pupils aged 10 or 11. Two pupils are preverbal and one is at a one word level. Pupils have symbol recognition skills. Two adults will work with the children.
Context	Speech and language therapist is joining the group for this session. This session has been ongoing for several weeks.
Approaches	Sensory approaches; Symbols.
Resources	Book such as *We're Going on a Bear Hunt*; chocolate and sprinkles (mud); box and black material (cave); water spray (river); shredded green paper (grass); icing sugar (snow); symbols.
Environment	Chairs in a circle facing the teacher. Trays are available for sensory materials. There is a felt board for large symbols but the book itself is not displayed as it will distract from eye contact/attention to the speaker. Resources are hidden behind a screen in order to avoid distraction. Session conducted in easy to clean location.
Content	- Intro. – 'Hello' to everyone. Children bang on drum to indicate their presence. - Two bears are presented. Each week a different child chooses which bear to use. - Adult starts to recite story. Other adult repeats line and encourages pupils to focus and join in with actions. - Symbols used to introduce each part of the story. Associated prop is given to pupils to touch. - If any child shows particular interest in a prop they can request the item using a symbol. They are then able to play with the item. - When the story is finished, children can use symbols to request a particular section again. - When the last child has chosen, count down from 10 is used to finish the lesson.
Contingency	Children to be allowed to leave the group if they don't want to participate.
Discussion	This is a lesson in which the manipulation of the **environment** is crucial to success. The focus of the session is active listening and participation, therefore, the book is not used; the speaker becomes the centre of attention. The **sensory needs** of the group are addressed by the use of resources. Note the use of the **countdown** to structure the end of the session.

Mathematics

Learning Objectives	• to take turns in the activity, • to sequence the events of the day, • to practise counting skills, and • to investigate the properties of 2-D shapes.
About the Group	Six pupils aged between five and seven years. All children with statements of SEN specifying ASDs compounded by SLD. One child using one word level, all other children preverbal. High staff to pupil ratio (3:6). All children display some degree of challenging behaviour. Varied personalities in the group balance each other well. Children are beginning to anticipate the routine of the lesson.
Context	Lesson delivered as part of regular daily circle time.
Approaches	TEACCH; PECS; Planned Behaviour Support.
Resources	Laminated visual aids; white magnetic board; tape recorder.
Environment	Children seated in semi-circle, facing display board. Cupboards and screens are used to block out distractions and define group area.
Content	• Photos/symbols (daily timetable) are passed around the group. • Each child places the photo/symbol on the board in the correct place. • One child counts the number of children present. • Each child places their own photo on maths board and then the group count how many children are present. • Shapes are laid out on floor. Each child has been given a shape and has to match their shape to the corresponding shape on the floor. Adult discusses number of sides, properties etc.
Contingency	All children are required to stay with the group throughout the session. If a child becomes significantly challenging they may be removed to another adult directed activity.
Discussion	There is an emphasis on highly **visual resources.** The familiarity of the daily routine is used to enable children to sequence events building on the characteristic **strengths** of the learner with autism. There is variation in the emphasis between **individual** and **group work** giving each child the opportunity to develop their skills within a supportive framework. The session is characterised by the **tangible** nature of the resources used. Children can make progress without relying on language skills.

Educating Pupils with Autistic Spectrum Disorders © Martin Hanbury, 2005

Science

Learning Objectives	• to investigate changes in materials.
About the Group	Five pupils aged between 12 and 14. Diverse ability from preverbal to Level 2. Challenging behaviour displayed by all pupils. Staff to pupil ratio of 3:5.
Context	Session related to termly topic of 'change' and part of regular timetable science lesson. Taught in pupils' classroom in order to provide stability and familiar surroundings. Group work limited to short sessions; class teacher aiming to extend the duration of these.
Approaches	TEACCH; PECS; Planned Behaviour Support.
Resources	Trays, digital camera, various ice shapes (cubes, balloons, lollies).
Environment	Typical TEACCH classroom with distinct work areas for group and individual work. Low distraction environment. Access to outside area. Relaxing music is usually played in the background to promote a calm atmosphere.
Content	• Pupils sit around table, groups spaced apart. Adult says, 'Time for science', supported by appropriate symbol. No further language will be used. • Empty trays distributed to group. Ice shapes shared amongst pupils. • Adults encourage investigation by physically prompting pupils to handle ice. • Digital camera is used to record lesson. • After approximately 15 minutes, more able child moves to individual work-station to download pictures of session and record findings in written form with adult support. • As ice melts, pupils are encouraged to play with melted water, adding food colouring, splashing etc. • As pupils lose interest or if play becomes too agitated, pupils redirected to independent activity. • Pupils allowed to play for up to 20 minutes before being redirected to new activity. • Lesson followed up with photographs the following day during group time.
Contingency	Lesson could be delivered using trays in individual work-stations if group work becomes difficult.
Discussion	This session is focused on **experiential** learning in order to develop understanding of complex scientific concepts. **No language** is used in order to enable the pupils to focus entirely on the content of the session without needing to process language. The **open-ended** conclusion of the lesson allows pupils to explore as far as they are able.

Educating Pupils with Autistic Spectrum Disorders © Martin Hanbury, 2005

PSHE

Learning Objectives	• to take responsibility for own behaviour, • to form associations between behaviour and the degree of independence achieved, and • to generalise self-advocacy skills.
About the Group	Two 10-year-old pupils currently educated apart from other children on a one-to-one basis due to challenging behaviour. Generally, the pupils are functioning at about Level 2 of the National Curriculum. The children are verbal, can communicate their thoughts and opinions and have some elementary advocacy skills.
Context	The pupils work together in their own classroom and with two members of staff selected specifically for this work.
Approaches	TEACCH; SPELL; Planned Behaviour Support.
Resources	Wipe boards and pens; visual information on worksheets.
Environment	Ultimate low arousal environment, clearly demarcated physical boundaries.
Content	• Intro. – show pictures of people of different ages (infant to young adult). • Discuss how range of choices increase with age, what those choices are and how this is communicated to a person. • Show how dangerous choices result in independence being restricted and how this differs from age group to age group. • Worksheet showing various situations considering emotional welfare and encouraging reflection and opinion. • Finish lesson by agreeing contract of behaviour.
Contingency	Pupils to work in separate rooms if unable to work together. If necessary abandon lesson until pupil is calm enough to complete task.
Discussion	This lesson is focused on the urgent need to enable these pupils to manage their own behaviour appropriately. It is **realistic** in that the lesson will be postponed if the pupil is too agitated to learn effectively, yet **persistent** in that the work will be revisited until it is completed. Essentially the pupils are **highly motivated** to succeed as progress in this area will enable them to access a degree of independence they are keen to achieve. Visual materials are used to focus the pupils and engage them in comparatively **abstract discussion** around a **tangible** resource, resulting in opportunities for peer interaction between the pupils.

Food Technology

Learning Objectives	• to develop life skills, • to encourage independence, and • to promote communication amongst peers.
About the Group	Seven pupils aged between nine and 11 working with four members of staff. It is a diverse group ranging from preverbal to verbal pupils; some with good motor skills and others who are still unable to write or use scissors. Some of the pupils have challenging behaviour.
Context	Lesson takes place in food technology room.
Approaches	PECS; SPELL; standing back as much as possible to allow pupils independence.
Resources	Ingredients; timer; symbol choice boards; sentence prompts; symbolic representation of recipes.
Environment	Kitchen area labelled with symbols; ingredients in a box. Not everything required is laid out so that pupils have to locate things themselves as necessary.
Content	• Pupils prompted to collect drink choices from peers. • Pupils to travel as independently as possible to food technology room. • Pupils to follow instructions presented in a range of ways including written instructions, symbol strips or simply reading the packet. • Range of drinks to be made such as green tea, milk shake, juice. • Pupils clear away and take drinks back to class group on a tray. • Whole group enjoy drinks together.
Contingency	Increase level of staff support if pupil is finding difficulties. Child to return to classroom if unable to remain calm. Liaison with family/carers to practise these skills at home.
Discussion	This activity is highly motivating to the pupils as the **reward** is obvious and integral to the task. All instruction is **supported visually** enabling staff to promote **independence** by minimal intervention. The clear sequence of beginning, middle and end to the lesson provides **structure** and security for the pupils. This lesson improves the child's **self-esteem** as they are able to transfer these skills to home, for example, providing drinks for the family.

Geography

Learning Objectives	• to recall a recent journey.
About the Group	A student in a further education setting working on a one to one basis with a member of staff. The student has limited verbal skills but has prior knowledge of using TEACCH and PECS.
Context	The student is in the second term at college. The student and member of staff have been on a nature walk and are discussing the walk.
Approaches	Verbal questions supported by the member of staff drawing visual prompts.
Resources	Pen; paper.
Environment	Calm quiet place seated at an uncluttered table.
Content	• Member of staff gives verbal encouragement to student to recall walk. • Member of staff signposts different stages of the walk saying, for example, 'Do you remember the blossom on the tree?' • Staff member then draws tree and blossom. • Moves onto next stage using direction arrows for turning right/left. • Eventually completes visual map of the nature walk to support student's recollection of events.
Contingency	If student hesitant in response, staff member to chose different cue to support recall.
Discussion	The technique used in the lesson is very straightforward and can be **generalised** to a range of different settings, particularly when **promoting independence.** For example, the use of a **visual map** might be used to enable a person to recall a bus journey so that they replicate it independently. Equally, this technique might be used to support a person's recollection of where items are in the home or workplace or in order to structure the way a person completes domestic tasks.

Physical Education

Learning Objectives	• to respond correctly to instructions, • to identify and explore space to work in, and • to investigate different ways of moving.
About the Group	Eight pupils aged between seven and eight, varying in ability from pupils with SLD to more able pupils with Asperger Syndrome. Some of the children have challenging behaviours. There are four members of staff present.
Context	Lesson is consistently set in the context of the day for the pupils and is part of their regular timetable. The lesson takes place in the gym.
Approaches	• Indirect Method – teacher demonstrates task, pupils practise without adult direction. • Direct Method – tasks are presented and pupils are directed through each stage by adult. • Limitation Method – pupils explore their own way to complete tasks set by teacher.
Resources	Purpose-built gym; mats; benches; trestles; different coloured hoops; parachute; cassette player and relaxation music.
Environment	Well lit, high ceiling room. Walls painted magnolia, sound diffusion panels. Floor marked for different sports, such as five-a-side or badminton.
Content	• Warm up – move freely around space, e.g. walking or jogging, according to instruction. Stop, sit, stand as instructed. Pupils given support as needed. • Scatter the floor with various coloured hoops. Pupils to run around and then respond to instruction to 'Stop! Find Red/Green/Yellow' etc. • Reduce number of hoops each time. • Divide group into three smaller groups for apparatus work. Allocate staff as necessary. • Groups to complete circuit of apparatus using differentiated skills, including 1) walking along and jumping off; 2) walking along, jumping off and sinking down; 3) walking along, jumping off, sinking down and forward roll. • End of session pupils help to put away equipment. • Parachute is used to refocus pupils. Each pupil holds the edge of the parachute and wafts it up and down. Each child encouraged to lie down under parachute whilst relaxing music is playing. Gradually fade out music. • Pupils return to changing room.
Contingency	Shorten or lengthen phases of lesson as necessary.
Discussion	The precise **structure** and range of instruction techniques provide a successful combination of flexibility and framework. The lesson is strongly visual; verbal instructions are supported by **modelling** and familiarity. Concluding with a **relaxation** session enables the pupils to return to their classroom calmly.

History

Learning Objectives	• to develop an understanding of sequenced events, and • to recognise episodes from their own life.
About the Group	Six pupils aged between 11 and 13. Ability ranges from one to three preverbal pupils with with two to three word understanding and reading at Level 1. Two of the pupils have challenging behaviour. Staff to pupil ratio is 3:6. The group have mathematical skills well in advance of their communication skills.
Context	Lesson is related to the termly topic 'Myself' and will form the basis of a permanent classroom display. Each family has sent photographs into school marking events from the child's life (birthdays, christening etc.). The display will be frequently referred to during group time in order to reinforce the learning objectives.
Approaches	TEACCH; PECS; Planned Behaviour Support.
Resources	Long roll of paper with timeline drawn on; personal photographs; scissors; glue.
Environment	Typical TEACCH classroom with distinct areas for group and individual work.
Content	• Pupils gather around group work table. Timeline is rolled out. • Pupils present their own photographs to the group, describing the event. Symbols are used to support this as necessary. • Pupils are encouraged to guess their age at the time of the event or to state whether they were a baby, a little girl/boy, an older girl/boy. • Each pupil in turn places their photos on the timeline. Sequence is critically discussed. Necessary changes are made to present correct sequence. • Final product is discussed. Photos secured to timeline. • Timeline is displayed.
Contingency	A timeline with numbers 1–10 has been prepared to enable pupils to sequence events without the need to process dates.
Discussion	This lesson draws on the strong **visual skills** of children with autism and the characteristic ability to find order and pattern. The personal photographs are **motivating** and the events they describe familiar. The lesson actively engages the pupils' **families** in their learning.

Music

Learning Objectives	• to participate in singing familiar songs, and • to play a beat on a percussion instrument following an adult model.
About the Group	Seven pupils aged between five and 12. The children in the group have very limited language skills; preverbal to one word level. Staff to pupil ratio is 4:7. Children recognise variety of PECS symbols.
Context	This group has been formed from across the school specifically for this set of music lessons conducted over the course of a school term.
Approaches	TEACCH; PECS; Planned Behaviour Support.
Resources	Guitar; variety of percussion instruments; CD and CD player.
Environment	The classroom has been divided in half using screens. In one half, percussion instruments are laid out on tables; in the other half, a space is cleared and chairs are formed in a circle. Soft background music is playing.
Content	• Children sit on chairs in circle; staff interspersed amongst pupils. • Leader greets everyone saying, 'Hello, it's time for music' and shows large music symbol to group. • Sing 'Hello song'. Leader plays guitar and directs greeting to each child. • Choose board with symbols for various songs ('Old MacDonald'; 'Row Your Boat' etc.) is offered to each child in turn. When all have chosen, board is put away. • Leader says, 'Time for instruments' and shows photograph of several percussion instruments. Children are directed into other half of classroom. • CD of strongly rhythmic music (e.g. Latin, African, Gamelan) is played. Children encouraged to pick up instruments and copy rhythms. Staff move around the room, modelling, encouraging, tapping out rhythms on child's body or dancing with a child. Session lasts maximum of 15 minutes. • Leader gives one minute warning of finish. CD is turned off. Children directed back to chairs. • Sing 'Goodbye song'.
Contingency	Each component of the lesson can be shortened or extended as necessary.
Discussion	Music provides children with autism **expressive** opportunities within a **natural structure**. This lesson focuses on group dynamics and then on individual expression. The **physicality** of music is explored. Note how a **warning** is given before the end of the 'free-style' session, reintroducing the directive element of the session gradually.

Educating Pupils with Autistic Spectrum Disorders © Martin Hanbury, 2005

Conclusion

We can affect nothing more than ourselves. In the field of ASDs, that is probably the most important change we can bring about. By making ourselves more effective practitioners, whether we are working in a mainstream, special or specialist setting, we will ultimately benefit the children with whom we are working.

Children with ASDs face many challenges; challenges they did not choose. We, on the other hand, have chosen the challenges we face in the field of autism and are therefore obliged to become as skilled and effective as possible in addressing those challenges. Over the last 20 years, we have made great progress in our knowledge, understanding and skill in the education of children with autism. It is the practitioner in the classroom who has achieved this and it is with the practitioner that future progress in the field lies. Good luck.

Glossary

aetiology – the root cause of a condition or disease

BILD – British Institute of Learning Disabilities

central coherence theory – the instinct to place information into a context, to look for the bigger picture

closed task – a task in which the outcome is predetermined wherein there is a right answer

DSM IV – Diagnostic and Statistical Manual (Edition 4)

epidemiological research – research which is concerned with the study of the prevalence of a condition

executive function – an in-built mechanism for analysing situations and selecting a course of action

functionally significant – behaviour which addresses a need a person has

GAP – Good Autism Practice

homographs – words which are spelt in the same way but differ in meaning

ICD 10 – International Classification of Diseases

INSET – IN-Service Training

learning planning meeting – a meeting held to share assessment information with parents and discuss objectives for the child's learning

mind-blindness – the inability to comprehend other people's mental states

NAPC – National Autism Plan for Children

NAS – National Autistic Society

neurochemicals – chemicals within the brain which regulate activity and transmit essential messages

open task – a task whose outcome is not pre-determined, in which success is determined by the quality of the process and product of the work rather than by a right or wrong answer

outreach – a range of support services focused on providing a continuum of support for children in mainstream settings

PECS – Picture Exchange Communication System

pica – eating non-food items such as soil, glue, paint

SPELL – Structure, Positive approaches and expectations, Empathy, Low arousal, Links

TEACCH – Treatment and Education of Autistic and related Communication handicapped CHildren

theory of mind – the ability to consider the thoughts, feelings and motives of another person

triad of impairments – difficulties experienced in all three areas of social understanding, social communication and imagination

Useful Organisations

The National Autistic Society
393 City Road, London, EC1V 1NG, UK
+44 (0)20 7833 2299
www.nas.org.uk

Pyramid Educational Consultants UK Ltd
Pavilion House, 6 Old Steine, Brighton, BN1 1EJ, UK
+44 (0)1273 609555
www.pecs.org.uk

Pyramid Educational Consultants Inc
226 West Park Place, Suite 1, Newark DE. 19711, USA
+1 888 732 7462
www.pecs.com

Division TEACCH
CB# 7180, 100 Renee Lynne Court,
The University of North Carolina at Chapel Hill
Chapel Hill, NC 27599-7180, USA
+1 919 966 2174
www.teacch.com

British Institute of Learning Disability
Campion House, Green Street, Kidderminster,
Worcestershire, DY10 1JL, UK
+44 (0)1562 723010
www.bild.org.uk

Good Autism Practice Journal
www.corelearning.co.uk/gap/

Bibliography

Aarons, M. and Gittens, T. (1992) *The Autistic Continuum: An Assessment and Intervention Schedule*. Windsor: NFER.

American Psychiatric Association. (1992) *Diagnostic and Statistical Manual of Mental Disorders – Fourth Edition*. Washington DC: American Psychiatric Association.

Asperger, H. (1944) 'Die autistichen psychopathen im kindesalter', *Archiv für Psychiatrie und Nervenkrankenheiten* (Autistic Psychopathy in Childhood), 117: 76–136.

Barnard, J., Broach, S., Potter, D. and Prior, A. (2002) *Autism in Schools: Crisis or Challenge*. London: National Autistic Society.

Baron-Cohen, S. (1990) 'Autism: a specific cognitive disorder of "mind-blindness"', *International Review of Psychiatry*, 2: 79–88.

Baron-Cohen, S.(1995) *Mindblindness: An Essay on Autism and Theory of Mind*. London: Bradford Books.

Bondy, A.S. and Frost, L. (2002) *A Picture's Worth: PECS and Other Visual Communication Strategies in Autism*. Bethesda: Woodbine House.

Campbell, R., Baron-Cohen, S. and Walker, J. (1995) 'Do people with autism show a whole face advantage in recognition of familiar faces and their parts? A test of central coherence theory.' Unpublished manuscript, University of London, Goldsmith's College.

Charman, T. and Care, P. (2004) *Mapping Autism Research*. London: National Autistic Society.

Cohen, D. and Volkmar, F. (1997) *Handbook of Autism and Pervasive Developmental Disorders*. New York: John Wiley.

Creak, M. (1964) 'Schizophrenic syndrome in childhood: further progress report of a working party', *Developmental Medicine and Child Neurology*, 6: 530–5.

Cumine, V., Leach, J. and Stevenson, G. (2000) *Autism in the Early Years: A Practical Guide*. London: David Fulton.

Dewart, H. and Summers, S. (1988) *The Pragmatic Profile of Early Communication Skills*. London: NFER-Nelson.

Elgar, S. and Wing, L. (1975) *Teaching Autistic Children*. London: NCSE and NSAC.

Frith, U. (1989) *Autism: Explaining the Enigma*. Oxford: Blackwell.

Frost, L.A. and Bondy, A.S. (1994) *PECS: The Picture Exchange Communication System - Training Manual*. Cherry Hill, NJ: Pyramid Educational Consultants.

Frost, L.A. and Bondy, A.S. (2002) *The Picture Exchange Communication System - Training Manual*. Newark, DE: Pyramid Educational Products.

Gillberg, C. (1984) 'Infantile autism and other child psychoses in a Swedish urban region: epidemiological aspects', *Journal of Child Psychology and Psychiatry*, 25: 35–43.

Gillberg, C. (1985) 'Asperger's Syndrome and recurrent psychosis: a case study', *Journal of Autism and Developmental Disorders*, 15 (4): 389–97.

Gillberg, C., Steffenburg, S. and Schaumann, H. (1991) 'Is autism more common now than ten years ago?', *British Journal of Psychiatry*, 158: 403–9.

Gray, C. (1994a) *The Social Story Book*. Arlington: Future Horizons.

— (1994b) *Comic Strip Conversations*. Arlington: Future Horizons.

Gray, C. and Leigh White, A. (2002) *My Social Stories Book*. London: Jessica Kingsley.

Happe, F. (1997) 'Central coherence and theory of mind', *British Journal of Developmental Psychology*, 15(1): 1–12.

Happe, F. (1994) *Autism: An Introduction to Psychological Theory*. London: UCL Press.

Jordan, R. and Powell, S. (1995) *Understanding and Teaching Children with Autism*. Chichester: John Wiley.

Kanner, L. (1943) 'Autistic disturbances of affective contact', *The Nervous Child*, 2: 217–50.

Kiernan, C. and Reid, B. (1987) *Pre-Verbal Communication Schedule*. London: NFER-Nelson.

Leslie, A. M. (1987) 'Pretence and representation: the origins of "theory of mind"', *Psychological Review*, 94: 412–26.

Lotter, V. (1966) 'Epidemiology of autistic conditions in young children: I. Prevalence', *Social Psychiatry*, 1: 124–37.

Mesibov, G. and Howley, M. (2003) *Accessing the Curriculum for Pupils with Autistic Spectrum Disorders*. London: David Fulton.

NIASA (2003) *National Autism Plan for Children*. London: National Autistic Society.

Nind, M. and Hewett, D. (1994) *Access to Communication: Developing the Basics of Communication with People with Severe Learning Difficulties through Intensive Interaction*. London: David Fulton.

Nind, M. and Hewett, D. (2001) *A Practical Guide to Intensive Interaction*. Kidderminster: BILD Publications.

Norman, D. and Shallice, T. (1980) 'Attention to action: willed and automatic control of behaviour', in R. Davidson, G. Schwartz and D. Shapiro (eds) *Consciousness and Self-regulation*, Vol. 4. New York: Plenum Press, pp. 1–18.

Potter, C. and Whittaker, C. (2001) *Enabling Communication in Children with Autism*. London: Jessica Kingsley.

Prevezer, W. (1990) 'Strategies for tuning into autism', *Therapy Weekly*, 4: 18 October.

Rimland, B. (1964) *Infantile Autism*. New York: Appleton-Century-Crofts.

Rutter, M. (1978) 'Diagnosis and definition of childhood autism', *Journal of Autism and Childhood Schizophrenia*, 8: 139–161.

Schopler, E., Reichler, R.J., Bashford, A., Lansing, M.D. and Marcus, L.M. (1990) *Psychoeducational Profile – Revised (PEP – R)*. Austin, TX: Pro-Ed.

Schopler, E. and Mesibov, G. (1995) *Learning and Cognition in Autism*. New York: Plenum Press.

Shah, A. and Frith, U. (1983) 'An islet of ability in autism: a research note,' *Journal of Child Psychology and Psychiatry* 34: 613–20.

Sherratt, D. and Peter, M. (2002) *Developing Play and Drama in Children with Autistic Spectrum Disorders*. London: David Fulton.

Sigman, M., Mundy, P., Ungerer, J. and Sherman, T. (1986) 'Social interactions of autistic, mentally retarded, and normal children and their caregivers', *Journal of Child Psychology and Psychiatry*, 27 (5): 647–56.

Wimpory, D. (1995) 'Brief Report: Musical interaction therapy for children with autism: an evaluative case study', *Journal of Autism and Developmental Disorders*, 25 (5): 541–52.

Wing, L. (1993) 'The definition and prevalence of autism: a review', *European Child and Adolescent Psychiatry*, 2 (2): 61–74.

Wing, L. (1996) *The Autistic Spectrum*. London: Constable and Robinson Ltd.

Wing, L. and Gould, J. (1979) 'Severe impairments of social interaction and associated abnormalities in children: epidemiology and classification', *Journal of Autism and Childhood Schizophrenia*, 9: 11–29.

Wing, L. and Potter, D. (2002) 'The epidemiology of autistic spectrum disorders: is prevalence rising?', *Mental Retardation and Developmental Disabilities Research Reviews*, 8 (3): 151–61.

World Health Organization. (1993) *Mental Disorders: A Glossary and Guide to their Classification in Accordance with the 10th Revision of the International Classification of Diseases (ICD-10)*. Geneva: World Health Organisation.

Index

Paul Chapman Publishing and Lucky Duck

Autism and Early Years Practice

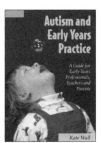

A Guide for Early Years Professionals, Teachers and Parents

Kate Wall *Canterbury Christ Church University College*

'A remarkable reference resource. It is, without a doubt, the most absorbing and easily absorbed book we have seen, setting out the most comprehensive survey of the history, definitions, needs of carers and sufferers, issues of diagnosis, and much, much more' - ***Nurturing Potential***

Written for the practitioner, this book offers useful, practical, realistic and constructive suggestions for early years practice - all supported by individual case studies as exemplars.

2004 • 184 pages
Cloth (1-4129-0127-8) / Paper (1-4129-0128-6)

Special Needs and Early Years

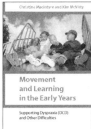

A Practitioner's Guide

Kate Wall *Canterbury Christ Church University College*

'This is one of the best books I have read on special needs and the very young and I thoroughly recommend it to all with a professional or personal interest in this area' - ***Special Children***

Kate Wall shares her expertise in this accessible book for practitioners. Based on her own research and practice, she covers such topics as working with families, partnerships with parents, observation and assessment, programmes of intervention, and responding to the affective needs of children.

2003 • 198 pages
Cloth (0-7619-4075-8) / Paper (0-7619-4076-6)

Movement and Learning in the Early Years

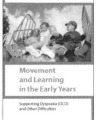

Supporting Dyspraxia (DCD) and Other Difficulties

Christine Macintyre *Freelance Consultant* and **Kim McVitty** *Nursery School Teacher*

'It is always good to be able to welcome a book on such a key factor as movement in early childhood development, and this text has been written to support parents and practitioners who wish to understand how movement contributes to all aspects of learning - intellectual, social and emotional, as well as physical' - ***Marian Whitehead, Nursery World***

This book shows you how to observe a child as they move to allow for early identification of any problems. It also tells you how to help with lots of suggested activities.

2004 • 160 pages
Cloth (1-4129-0236-3) / Paper (1-4129-0237-1)

From Another Planet

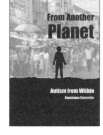

Autism from Within

Dominique Dumortier

When they read this book my friends and acquaintances may not immediately recognise it is about me. I have become an expert at hiding difficulties caused by my autism.

This book explains the experience of the author, Dominique Dumortier, facing the everyday events we easily manage. It helps us understand the condition, anticipate the problems that arise and respond with flexibility and acceptance.

Lucky Duck Books
2004 • 112 pages
Paper (1-904315-32-1)

Aspects of Asperger's

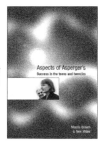

Success in the Teens and Twenties

Maude Brown and **Alex Miller**

This thought provoking and practical book looks at how one supporter - a grandmother - helped her granddaughter search for ways to overcome the difficulties they both faced. Useful to all those whose lives are touched by Asperger's Syndrome, it is especially meaningful to those directly involved in supporting young people in school, college and in the home and neighbourhood setting.

Lucky Duck Books
2004 • 82 pages
Paper (1-904315-12-7)

Martian in the Playground

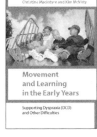

Understanding the Schoolchild with Asperger's Syndrome

Clare Sainsbury

WINNER OF TES/NASEN BEST ACADEMIC BOOK AWARD 2000

'It is to be hoped that teachers and others who deal with children and young people in group settings will read this book and realize that there is a positive as well as a negative side to autism' - ***Jane Lovey, Cambridge University School of Education***

This exceptional book illuminates what it means to be a person who has Asperger's Syndrome by providing a window into a unique and particular world.

Lucky Duck Books
2000 • 140 pages
Paper (1-87394-208-7)

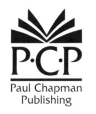

P·C·P
Paul Chapman
Publishing

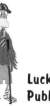

**Lucky Duck
Publishing**

Order online at www.PaulChapmanPublishing.co.uk